58.50

369 0240860

A Guide to Neonatal and Pediatric ECGs

Maria Albina Galli • Gian Battista Danzi

A Guide to Neonatal and Pediatric ECGs

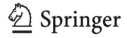 Springer

Maria Albina Galli
Division of Cardiology
Section of Perinatal and
Pediatric Cardiology
Fondazione IRCCS Ca' Granda
Ospedale Maggiore Policlinico
University of Milan
Milan, Italy

Gian Battista Danzi
Cardiologist
Milan, Italy

Originally published as
Guida all'ECG neonatale e pediatrico, by Maria Albina Galli and Gian Battista Danzi
© 2010 Il Pensiero Scientifico Editore

ISBN 978-88-470-2855-5   ISBN 978-88-470-2856-2 (eBook)

DOI 10.1007/978-88-470-2856-2

Springer Milan Dordrecht Heidelberg London New York

Library of Congress Control Number: 2012954886

© Springer-Verlag Italia 2013

9 8 7 6 5 4 3 2 1   2013 2014 2015 2016

Cover design: Ikona S.r.l., Milan, Italy
Typesetting: Graphostudio, Milan, Italy

Springer-Verlag Italia S.r.l. – Via Decembrio 28 – I-20137 Milan
Springer is a part of Springer Science+Business Media (www.springer.com)

To my parents and my aunts, Elena and Anna
Maria Albina Galli

Preface

This manual is meant for cardiologists, pediatricians, neonatologists, pediatric cardiac surgeons, emergency medicine physicians, nursing personnel, medical students and residents who possess the basic knowledge to read an ECG and need to know the specific procedures to apply to pediatrics.

This manual provides a highly simplified method for pediatric ECG analysis. It requires observing only a few elements but allows for the immediate recognition of a pathological condition.

Part I delineates the ECG reading method to follow, as well as describing normal pediatric ECG parameters. Part II provides a description of pathological scenarios specific to pediatrics. Finally, in Part III, the manual provides the most common applications for pediatric ECGs.

Milan, December 2012   Maria Albina Galli

Contents

Part I
Normal ECGs

1

The pediatric ECG reading method is based on the fact that the morphology of a normal ECG varies with age. The electrical activity of the heart reflects hemodynamic cardiac changes, which are at their height in the first month of life and which continue, in part, through the first year of life and beyond.

The general guideline is: a normal pediatric ECG is one in which the morphology is congruous with the age of the young patient. Attention must be paid to the morphology of ventricular depolarization (the QRS complex) and of ventricular repolarization (the T wave). The morphology of these two elements, which change mainly during the first few months of life, should be in accordance with the age of the patient.

Three patterns can be distinguished through the morphology of the QRS complex and the T wave:
- The neonatal pattern.
- The infant pattern.
- The adult pattern.

The neonatal pattern ECG is typical in the first month of life. In a normal subject, this changes after the first month and takes on the characteristics of the infant pattern, which can last up to the age of three. After this point, it changes again, taking on the characteristics of the adult pattern.

Normally, the ECG pattern is in line with the age of the patient. Finding an ECG pattern that is incongruous with the patient's age, for example a neonatal pattern after the first month of life, leads to the conclusion that there is pathological reason. Thus, a series of ECGs conducted on the same patient over time can be very useful to pinpoint the emergence of pathological signs.

It is useful to specify that the terms "newborn" and "infant" are not equivalent to the "neonatal" and "infant" ECG patterns. There is a temporal correspondence between a "newborn", i.e. a child in the first month of life, and a "neonatal ECG pattern", which occurs only in the first month of life for normal subjects. This is not the case, however, for the term "infant", referring to a child in the first year of life, and the term "infant ECG pattern", which can occur at birth and last until the age of three.

1.1 The Neonatal Pattern

A normal ECG from birth and through the first month of life has some characteristics that identify it as the "neonatal pattern". The neonatal pattern shows prevalent electrical

M. A. Galli (✉)
Perinatal and Pediatric Cardiology
Ospedale Maggiore Policlinico
Milan, Italy
e-mail: mariellagalli@gmail.com

M. A. Galli, G. B. Danzi, *A Guide to Neonatal and Pediatric ECGs*,
DOI: 10.1007/978-88-470-2856-2_1, © Springer-Verlag Italia 2013

Table 1.1 Neonatal pattern. Ventricular depolarization. The electrical prevalence of the right ventricle is the norm for newborns

QRS – Neonatal pattern	
In V_1 R wave dominates in that R/S > 1	(R/S ratio: from 1 to 7)
	(R wave < 25 mm)
	(S wave < 20 mm)
In V_6: S wave dominates in that R/S < 1	(S wave < 10 mm)
In V_1: if R wave is exclusive	< 13 mm in the 1st week of life
	< 10 mm after 1st week of life

activity in the right ventricle. This prevalence is normal for newborns since it resembles the hemodynamic condition of a fetus. After the 31st week of gestation until term, the right ventricle of the fetus gains myocardial mass because it pumps against the high resistance of the small muscular pulmonary arteries. The left ventricle, on the other hand, pumps against the low resistance of the placenta's blood vessels. At birth the mass difference between the right and left ventricles is a ratio of 1 to 1.3.

To define the neonatal pattern, two factors present in precordial leads are considered: 1) depolarizing electrical ventricular activity, that is the morphology of the QRS complex; and 2) repolarizing activity, that is the morphology of the T wave. It is sufficient to simply focus on two precordial leads: V_1 and V_6.

The V_1 precordial lead is the one facing the right ventricle. Thus, in the QRS complex, the R wave (the positive deflection) represents the depolarizing electrical activity of the right ventricle. Meanwhile, the S wave (the negative deflection) represents the depolarizing electrical activity of the left ventricle.

The V_6 precordial lead is the one facing the left ventricle. Thus in the QRS complex, the R wave (the positive deflection) corresponds to the depolarizing electrical activity of the left ventricle. Meanwhile, the S wave (the negative deflection) represents the depolarizing electrical activity of the right ventricle.

Since the electrical activity of the right ventricle prevails in the first month of life, the normal neonatal ECG pattern shows the prevalence of the electrical forces of the right ventricle. In the V_1 precordial lead the R wave

is dominant over the S wave in that R/S > 1 (the R wave in V_1 represents the depolarizing electrical activity of the right ventricle). In the V_6 precordial lead the S wave is dominant over the R wave in that R/S < 1 (the S wave in V_6 represents the depolarizing electrical activity of the right ventricle). In V_1, the R wave can be exclusive, but its voltage should be less than 13 mm (1.3 mV) in the first week of life and 10 mm (1 mV) afterwards (see Table 1.1).

With regards to repolarizing ventricular electrical activity, that is the morphology of the T wave, the neonatal pattern in the first week of life can have positive or negative T waves in V_1 and positive T waves in V_6, but a flat or negative T wave in V_6 should be considered at the limits of the norm. After the first week of life the neonatal pattern requires the T wave to be negative in the V_1 and V_2 precordial leads and positive in V_6 (see Table 1.2).

A positive T wave in V_1 after the first week of life should be regarded with suspicion and investigated because it has been used to indicate right ventricular hypertrophy. In fact, changes in the T wave in V_1–V_2 are correlated with systolic pressure in the right ventricle and thus correlate with changes in pulmonary vascular resistance (PVR). A positive T wave after the first week of life suggests PVR is

Table 1.2 Neonatal pattern. Ventricular repolarization

T WAVE – Neonatal pattern
In the 1st week of life:
• In V_1: positive/diphasic/negative T wave
• In V_6: positive/ flat/ negative T wave
After 1st week of life:
• In V_1 – V_2: negative T wave
• In V_6: positive T wave

still elevated. Elevated PVR is normal in the first week of life but afterwards it gradually reduces toward normal levels in normal subjects. A negative T wave shows normal maturation of the pulmonary vascular bed.

After the first week of life a positive T wave in V_1–V_2, indicates raised systolic pressure in the right ventricle, and can be a sign of congenital heart disease causing right ventricular pressure load.

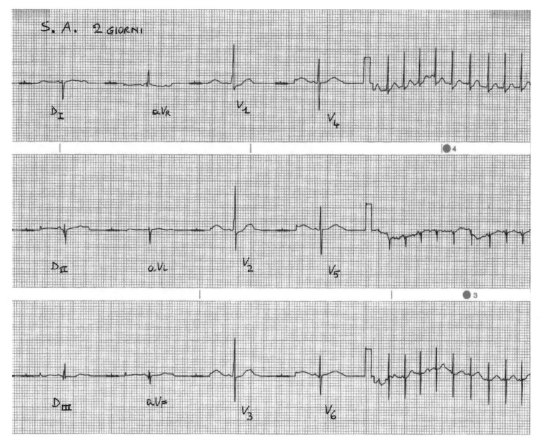

Fig. 1.1 Electrocardiogram recorded of a 2-day-old newborn

The ECG in Fig. 1.1 shows the characteristics of the "neonatal pattern". Looking at the morphology of the V_1 and V_6 precordial leads, one can see the prevalence of the right ventricle in ventricular depolarization (in V_1: R wave > S wave, therefore R/S > 1; in V_6: S wave is 8 mm deep, and R/S = 1). In the repolarizing electrical activity one can see a positive T wave in V_1–V_2 and V_6, fitting the normal pattern for the first week of life.

This patient was two days old and this "neonatal pattern" is congruous with his age, thus this ECG is normal.

The other parameters to be read are within the normal range defined in this manual: sinus rhythm, a PR interval of 100 ms, QRS duration of 50 ms, QRS frontal axis of +180° (strain and right axial deviation, which is normal in the first week of life), QTc interval of 452 ms (longer than the 440 ms normal limit, but not considered pathological in the first few weeks of life).

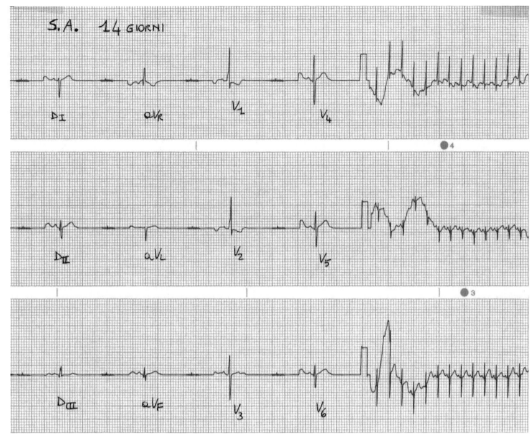

Fig. 1.2 Electrocardiogram of the same newborn as in Fig. 1.1, recorded at 14 days

   Considering the morphology of the V_1 and V_6 precordial leads, the trace in Fig. 1.2 maintains the characteristics of the "neonatal pattern" in terms of ventricular depolarization. It also shows the repolarizing electrical activity of the ventricles is evolving normally since the T wave changes from positive to negative in V_1–V_2 leads, as is normal after the first week of life. This signifies normal maturation of the pulmonary vascular bed, with gradual reduction of PVR. The QTc value of 433 ms has also normalized.

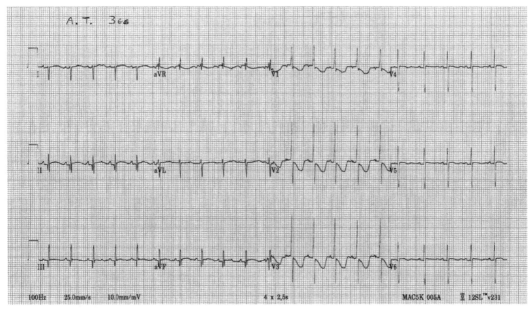

Fig. 1.3 Electrocardiogram recorded of a 3-day-old newborn

Characteristics of the "neonatal pattern" can be recognized in Fig. 1.3. In V_1, the R wave > the S wave therefore R/S > 1 and in V_6 the S wave is deep and has a voltage at the upper limits of the norm (1 mV) such that R/S < 1. The T wave of ventricular repolarization is negative in V_1, V_2 and V_3 precordial leads while it is flat in V_5 and V_6, which is a normal variant in the first week of life. The QRS frontal axis is right deviated (+140°) which is also normal in the first week of life. This electrocardiogram is normal since it is congruous with the age of the patient.

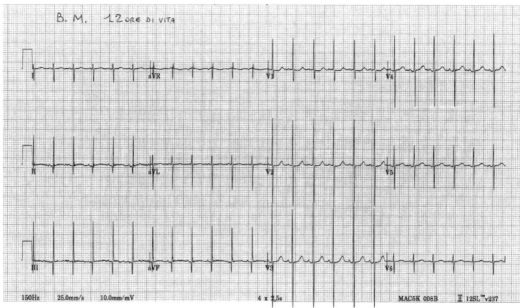

Fig. 1.4 Electrocardiogram recorded of a 12-hour-old newborn

In Fig. 1.4, with reference to ventricular depolarization (the V_1 and V_6 precordial leads), it is clear that the right ventricle electrical activity prevails, which is normal in the first month of life. The T wave of ventricular repolarization is positive in V_1–V_2, which is within the norm for the first week of life. The T wave is positive in V_5 and V_6, which is also normal. The QRS frontal axis is right deviated at +110°, which is within the norm through the first year of life. This ECG is normal because of the concordance between the "neonatal pattern" and the age of the patient, both in terms of depolarization and ventricular repolarization.

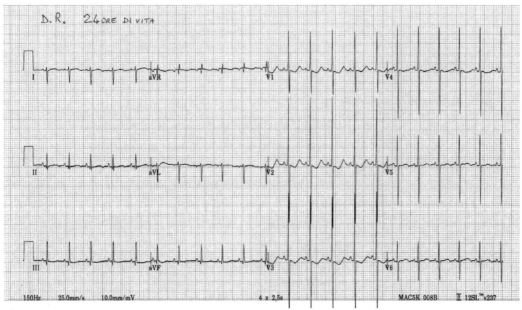

Fig. 1.5 Electrocardiogram recorded of a 24-hour-old newborn

In Fig. 1.5, the electrical prevalence of the right ventricle fits the "neonatal pattern" (in V_1 the R/S ratio > 1; in V_6 the R/S ratio = 1). In terms of ventricular repolarization, the T wave is diphasic in V_1, V_2 and V_3 (considered normal in the first week of life) and positive in V_5–V_6. All these elements indicate this trace is normal. The QRS frontal axis is right deviated at +120°, which is normal in relation to the patient's age.

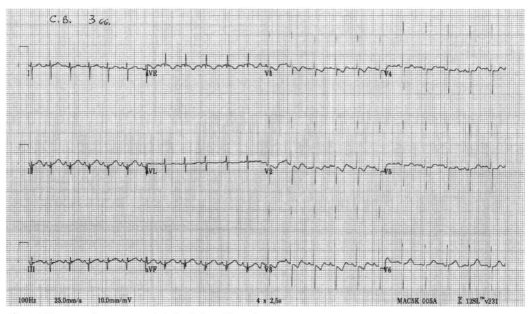

Fig. 1.6 Electrocardiogram recorded of a 3-day-old newborn

Looking at the V_1 and V_6 precordial leads in Fig. 1.6, one sees the electrical prevalence of the right ventricle, which fits the "neonatal pattern" and is congruous with the age of this 3-day-old patient. The morphology of ventricular repolarization already shows the normal reduction of the PVR since the T wave is negative in the V_1–V_2–V_3 precordial leads. The QRS frontal axis shows strain and right deviation (+180°), which is within the variations of the norm in the first week of life.

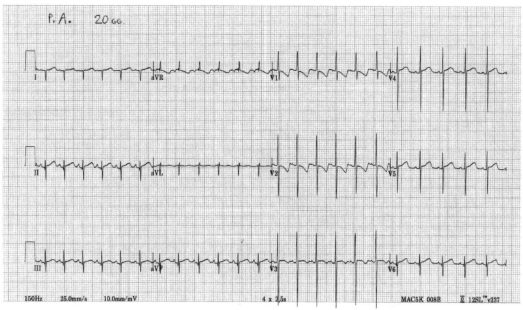

Fig. 1.7 Electrocardiogram recorded of a 20-day-old newborn

Figure 1.7 shows that, with regard to ventricular depolarization, the electrical forces in the right ventricle dominate both in V_1, in that R/S > 1, and in V_6 in that R/S < 1. In ventricular repolarization, the T wave is negative in V_1, V_2 and V_3 precordial leads and positive in V_5, and V_6. The QRS frontal axis has kept a strong right deviation at +170°, which is still to be considered within normal limits in the first month of life. All these elements fit the "neonatal pattern". These elements are appropriate for the age of the patient and this trace is interpreted as normal.

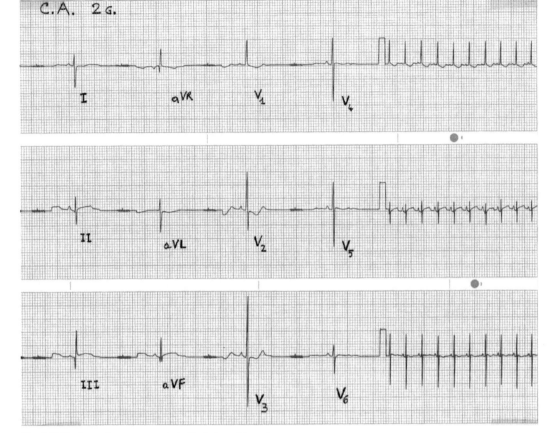

Fig. 1.8 Electrocardiogram recorded of a 2-day-old newborn

The ECG in Fig. 1.8 shows a variant of the "neonatal pattern" since the R wave is exclusive in V_1 (the S wave of electrical activity in the left ventricle is absent). For this to be normal, the voltage of the R wave must be less than 13 mm (1.3 mV) in the first week of life and less than 10 mm (1 mV) afterwards. In this case, the voltage of the exclusive R wave is 1 mV, so it is normal.

One can see that the electrical forces of the right ventricle are prevalent in V_6 such that R/S < 1. This is prescribed by the "neonatal pattern".

With reference to ventricular repolarization, the T wave is diphasic in V_1, V_2 and V_3, and flat or tendentially positive in V_5–V_6, which is a variant of the norm for the first week of life. The QRS frontal axis is right deviated at +150°, which is normal in the first week of life.

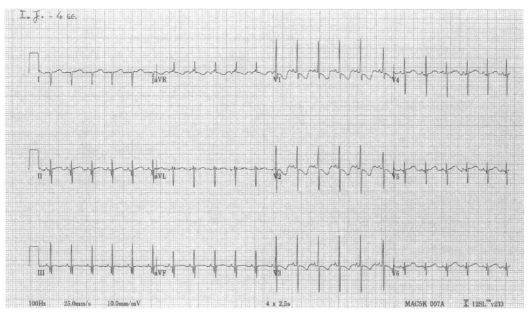

Fig. 1.9 Electrocardiogram recorded of a 4-day-old newborn

In the V_1 precordial lead in Fig. 1.9, a dominant depolarizing R wave of the right ventricle is visible such that R/S > 1. In V_6, one can see a depolarizing S wave of the right ventricle, which is dominant over the R wave of left ventricular depolarization such that R/S < 1. This confirms a morphology of electrical dominance of the right ventricle. This fits the "neonatal pattern" and is in concordance with the age of the patient, thus the ECG is normal. The ventricular repolarization is also normal since the T wave is negative in V_1–V_2–V_3 and positive in V_5–V_6 precordial leads.

The QRS frontal axis is right deviated at +160°, which is normal in the first week of life.

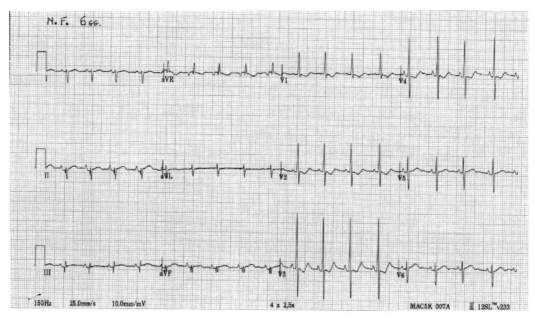

Fig. 1.10 Electrocardiogram recorded of a 6-day-old newborn

   In examining the morphology of ventricular depolarization in the precordial leads in Fig. 1.10, one can see the characteristics of the "neonatal pattern" of the right ventricular prevalence in electrical activity (in V_1, R/S > 1; in V_6, R/S < 1). As far as ventricular repolarization is concerned, the T wave is diphasic in V_1, V_2 and V_3 (normal in the first week of life) and positive in V_5–V_6. These elements mean this ECG is normal, since they are in concordance with this 6-day-old patient's age.

   The QRS frontal axis is extremely right deviated at +210°, which is still within normal limits for the first week of life.

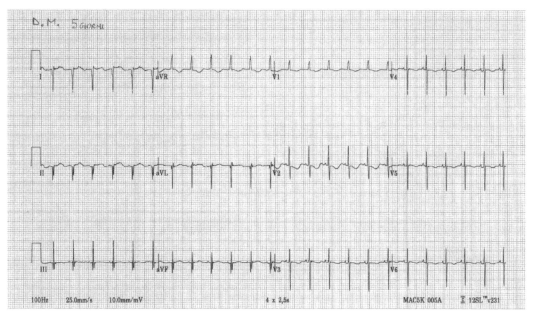

Fig. 1.11 Electrocardiogram recorded of a 5-day-old newborn

With regard to ventricular depolarization in the V_1 and V_6 precordial leads, one can see the "neonatal pattern" of right ventricular electrical dominance (Fig. 1.11), which is congruous with the age of the patient. In V_1, a 5 mm exclusive R wave is present, which is within the 1.3 mV normal limit for the first week of life. In V_6, the S wave of right ventricular depolarization prevails such that R/S < 1.

In terms of the morphology of ventricular repolarization, a negative T wave is observed in V_1, V_2 and V_3 as is normal. In V_6, the T wave is negative, which is a variant of the norm for the first week of life.

The QRS frontal axis is extremely right deviated at +210°, which is within the normal limits for the first week of life. This ECG is, therefore, normal in relation to the age of the patient.

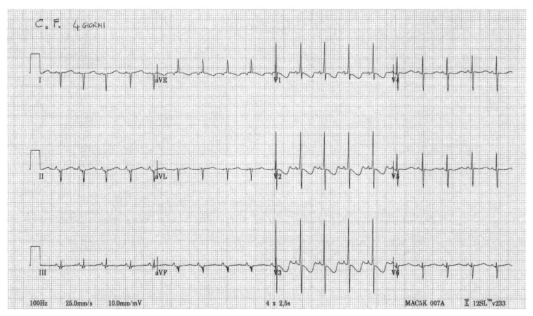

Fig. 1.12 Electrocardiogram recorded of a 4-day-old newborn

When considering ventricular depolarization, the "neonatal pattern" can be seen in the precordial leads V_1 and V_6 (Fig. 1.12), which is congruous with the age of the patient. The electrical force of the right ventricle prevails in V_1, with a dominant R wave such that R/S > 1. In V_6, the electrical force of the right ventricle still prevails, with a dominant S wave such that R/S < 1.

The morphology of ventricular repolarization fits the normal pattern since the T wave is negative in V_1, V_2 and V_3, and positive in V_6. The QRS frontal axis is right hyperdeviated at +200°, which is considered within the norm for the first week of life. This ECG is normal given the age of the patient.

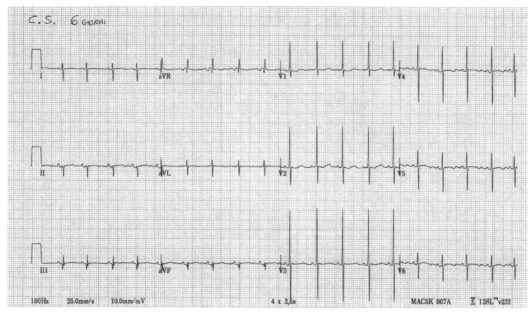

Fig. 1.13 Electrocardiogram recorded of a 6-day-old newborn

The "neonatal pattern" can also be recognized in Fig. 1.13, and is congruous with the age of the patient. In V_1, the electrical force of the right ventricle prevails, with a dominant R wave such that R/S > 1. In V_6, the electrical force of the right ventricle still prevails, with a dominant S wave such that R/S < 1.

With regard to ventricular repolarization, the T wave is still positive in V_1, V_2 and V_3, which is a variant of the norm in the first week of life. In V_6, the T wave is positive.

The QRS frontal axis is right hyperdeviated at +210°, which is normal for the first week of life. This ECG is normal considering the age of the patient.

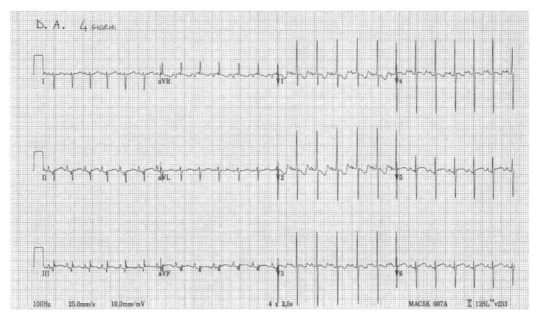

Fig. 1.14 Electrocardiogram recorded of a 4-day-old newborn

The "neonatal pattern" is well represented by the electrical dominance of the right ventricle in Fig. 1.14. In V_1, the R wave of the right ventricular depolarization prevails such that R/S > 1. In V_6, the S wave of right ventricular depolarization still prevails such that R/S < 1.

The morphology of ventricular repolarization is normal with a negative T wave in V_1, V_2 and V_3, and a positive one in V_6. The right hyperdeviation of the QRS frontal axis (+210°) is within the norm for the first week of life. Put together, these elements define this ECG as normal, given the age of the patient.

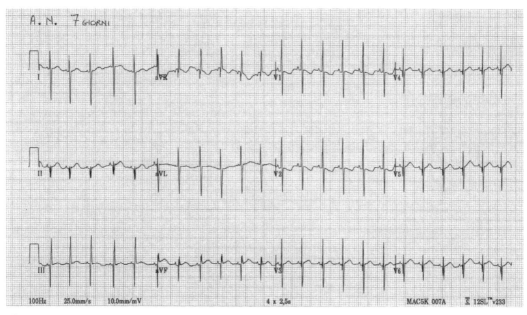

Fig. 1.15 Electrocardiogram recorded of a 7-day-old newborn

The electrical dominance of the right ventricle in the V_1 and V_6 precordial leads in Fig. 1.15 fits the "neonatal pattern". There are narrow and deep Q waves in the II, III and aV_F extremity leads. This aspect is a normal variation since the voltage is under 1 mV.

Ventricular repolarization is normal since the T wave is negative in V_1-V_2 and positive in V_6. The QRS frontal axis is right hyperdeviated at +200°, which is a variant of the norm in the first week of life. Therefore, this ECG is normal considering the age of the patient.

1.2   The Infant Pattern

Within the first few hours after birth hemodynamic changes begin, which form the basis of the morphological changes in the ECG.

The main change deals with PVR. A process of remodeling or maturation of the pulmonary vascular bed begins at birth. Over several months, the changes, which are at first dynamic, and later, anatomical, bring about the hemodynamic adult state.

At birth, a reduction in PVR begins because of:

• Dilation of the pulmonary muscular arterioles, mainly governed by a rise in partial oxygen pressure that comes with the onset of breathing and other vasodilating factors (prostacyclin I2, nitric oxide). Furthermore, vasoconstrictor effects of vasoactive mediators (hypoxia, acidosis, endothelin, thromboxane) become less effective.

• Recruitment of peripheral arteries previously closed in the fetal life, due to the draining of liquid that filled the alveoli (during gestation) and compressed the pulmonary vascular bed.

• Gradual decrease of medial muscle layer of the pulmonary arteries and arterioles by remodeling (lengthening and compression) of smooth muscle cells of the tunica media, with the consequent widening of the internal diameter of the vessel lumen and thinning of the tunica media in most of the distal muscular pulmonary arteries.

• Widening of the diameter of the small pulmonary arteries following the increase in pulmonary blood flow after birth.

The increase of the pulmonary vascular bed, and the gradual fall that results in PVR, bring about a gradual reduction in right ventricular systolic pressure. Consequently, right ventricular mass and right ventricular electrical forces gradually decrease.

After birth, the left ventricle follows the opposite course. It ceases to pump against the low resistance of the blood vessels in the placenta, and begins pumping against the high resistance of the peripheral blood vessels.

This brings about a rise in left ventricular systolic pressure and a gradual rise in left ventricular mass, which in turn raises the electrical force of the left ventricle.

Therefore, from birth through the first month of life, the right ventricle loses mass and electrical force through the gradual reduction of PVR. Meanwhile, the left ventricle gradually gains mass and electrical force by pumping against high peripheral vascular resistance. This dynamic continues and builds on itself throughout the first year of life. With the normalization of PVR and its systolic pressure, the right ventricle grows more slowly than the left. This is reflected in the relationship between the electrical forces of the two ventricles.

This gradual evolution, which reflects hemodynamic changes, balances the electrical forces of the left and right ventricles. This change marks the transfer from the "neonatal pattern" to what is defined as the "infant pattern". The "infant pattern" is characterized by balanced ventricular electrical forces. This is the normal ECG pattern found after the first month of life up to two years. Normal variants include the presence of this pattern already at birth all the way through to the age of 3.

Like in the "neonatal pattern", to define "the infant pattern" one must consider the morphology of the QRS complex and that of the T wave in the precordial leads. As with the neonatal pattern, it is sufficient to focus on V_1 and V_6. The positioning of the leads and the electrical activity indicated by the R and S waves are the same as described for the neonatal pattern.

After the first month of life the electrical forces of the ventricles are balanced, therefore, the infant ECG pattern shows equal electrical weight of the two ventricles. In the V_1 lead, the R wave will still be dominant over the S wave such that R/S > 1 (the R wave in V_1 represents the depolarizing electrical activity of the right ventricle), although to be considered normal, its voltage should be less than 20 mm (2 mV). In the V_6 precordial lead, the R wave will be dominant over the S wave

Table 1.3 Infant pattern. Ventricular depolarization. Balanced electrical forces in the ventricles are normal in infant pattern

QRS – Infant pattern	
In V_1: dominant R wave such that R/S > 1	R wave < 20 mm
In V_6: dominant R wave such that R/S > 1	R wave < 25 mm
	S wave < 10 mm
In V_1: if R wave is exclusive	R < 10 mm; never occurs after 1st year of life
In II–III–aV_F–V_6: Q wave up to 10 mm in depth	

Table 1.4 Infant pattern. Ventricular repolarization

T wave – Infant pattern	
In V_1–V_2–V_3: negative	after the 1st week of life up to age 8–10
In V_6: positive	after the 1st week of life

such that R/S > 1 (the R wave in V_6 represents the depolarizing electrical activity of the left ventricle), although to be considered normal, its voltage should be less than 25 mm (2.5 mV) and that of the S wave should be less than 10 mm (1 mV). In V_1, the R wave may be exclusive but to remain within the norm, its voltage should be less than 10 mm (1 mV) and never present after the first year of life (see Table 1.3).

A unique characteristic of the "infant pattern" is the potential for a narrow Q wave, up to 10 mm (1 mV) deep to appear in the II, III and aV_F extremity leads, as well as in the V_6 precordial lead. When this occurs, it is within the variations of the norm.

The "infant pattern" of the repolarizing electrical activity of the ventricles, has a negative T wave in V_1–V_2–V_3, as late as the age of 8–10 years and positive T wave in V_6 (see Table 1.4).

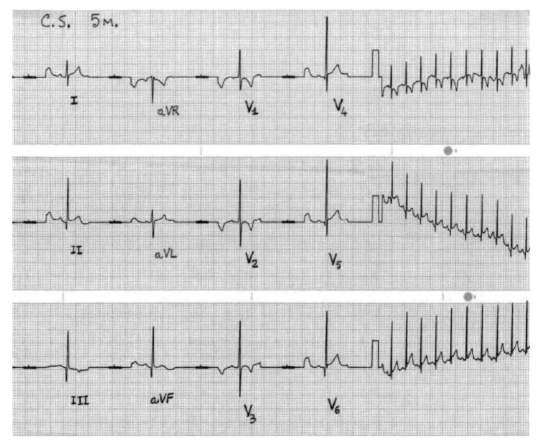

Fig. 1.16 Electrocardiogram recorded of a 5-month-old infant

This trace (Fig. 1.16) shows the characteristics of the "infant pattern". The morphology of the V_1 and V_6 precordial leads shows balanced electrical ventricular forces in ventricular depolarization (in V_1 the R wave is dominant such that R/S > 1; the expression of the right ventricular electrical forces is still strong. In V_6, the dominant R wave, the expression of the left ventricular electrical forces, is increasing). In ventricular repolarization, the T wave is negative in V_1, V_2 and V_3, and positive in V_5 and V_6. This is within the norm after the first week of life.

This patient is 5 months old and this "infant ECG pattern" is congruent with his age, so the trace is normal. The other parameters of interpretation are in line with the normal range defined in this guide: sinus rhythm, a PR interval of 120 ms, a QRS duration of 60 ms, a QRS frontal axis of +70°, a QTc interval of 398 ms.

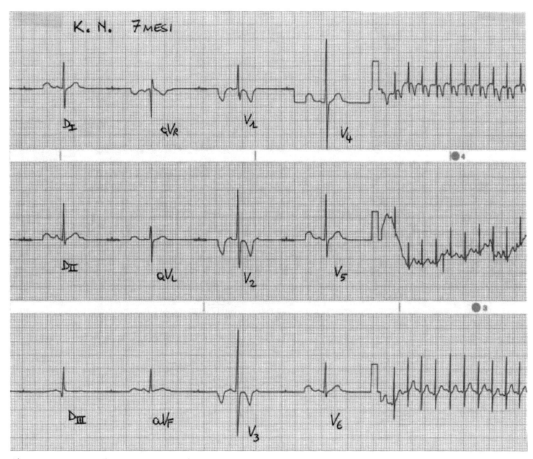

Fig. 1.17 Electrocardiogram recorded of a 7-month-old infant

In Fig. 1.17, for ventricular depolarization, one can see balanced ventricular electrical forces in the V_1 and V_6 precordial leads. In terms of ventricular repolarization, the T wave is negative in V_1, V_2 and V_3 and positive in V_5 and V_6. These qualities define the "infant pattern", which is appropriate for the age of this patient, thus this trace is normal.

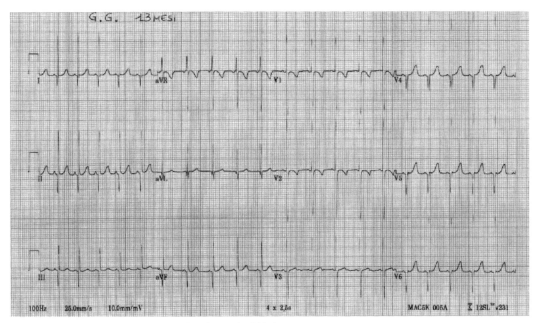

Fig. 1.18 Electrocardiogram recorded of a 13-month-old infant

In Fig. 1.18, for V_1, both the right ventricular depolarizing R wave and the left ventricular depolarizing S wave have almost equally high voltage, which is still within normal limits (2 mV). In V_6, the electrical activity of the left ventricle is dominant, with the S wave practically absent. All in all, one can say the electrical forces of the ventricles are balanced in this trace (Fig. 1.18), so it fits the "infant pattern". The "infant pattern" is characterized here by a deep Q wave in II, III, aV_F and V_6 leads, which does not surpass 10 mm (1 mV) in voltage and, thus is considered normal. In ventricular repolarization, the T wave is negative in V_1–V_2 and positive in V_5–V_6, which is normal. This ECG is appropriate for the age of the patient and is considered normal.

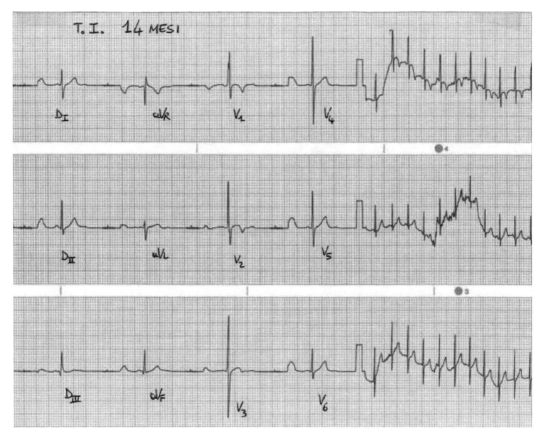

Fig. 1.19 Electrocardiogram recorded of a 14-month-old infant

In Fig. 1.19, with V_1, the R wave (electrical forces of the right ventricle) is dominant over the S wave with a slight slurring in the rise, an expression of brief delay in right intraventricular conduction, which should be considered a variant of the norm. In V_6, the R wave (electrical forces of the left ventricle) dominates over the S wave such that R/S > 1. These qualities indicate balanced electrical forces of the right and left ventricles, that is, an "infant pattern", congruent with the age of the patient. Ventricular repolarization is as it should be (T wave negative in V_1–V_2 and positive in V_5–V_6) and, at +80°, the QRS frontal axis is within the norm. This ECG is read as normal.

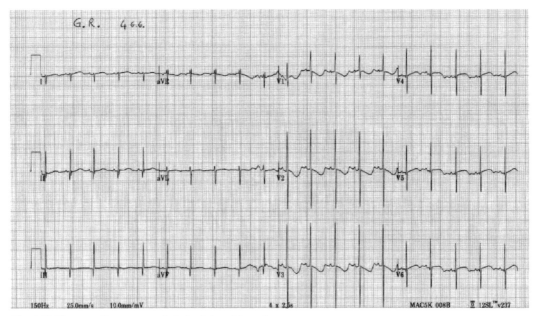

Fig. 1.20 Electrocardiogram recorded of a 4-day-old newborn

In Fig. 1.20, for V_1, the R wave (electrical forces of the right ventricle) is dominant over the S wave, and in V_6, the R wave (expression of electrical forces in the left ventricle) is dominant over the S wave, producing a situation with balanced ventricular electrical forces. This "infant pattern" can already be present at birth, so this electrocardiogram of a 4-day-old newborn should be considered normal. The normal morphology of ventricular repolarization (T wave negative in V_1, V_2 and V_3, and positive in V_5 and V_6) also confirms this ECG is normal.

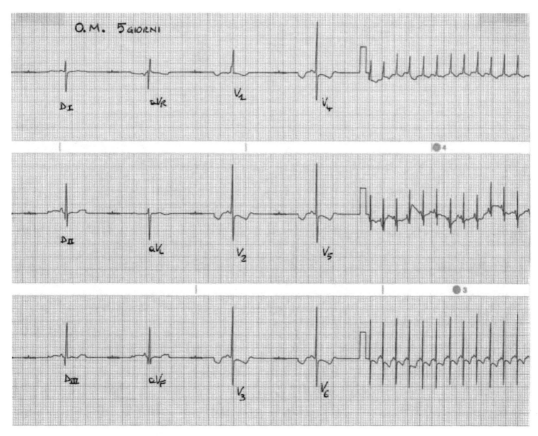

Fig. 1.21 Electrocardiogram recorded of a 5-day-old newborn

Here, a situation analogous to the one in Fig. 1.20 is shown. In this trace (Fig. 1.21), the electrical forces of the ventricles are balanced, thus this is an "infant pattern", which is considered normal even in the first week of life. The right ventricle's electrical dominance in V_1 is shown here by the exclusive 9 mm (0.9 mV) voltage R wave, which is within the 13 mm (1.3 mV) limit recommended for the first week of life. In V_6, the electrical dominance of the left ventricle is shown by the typical R/S > 1 relationship.

The morphology of ventricular repolarization is to be considered normal due to the negative T wave in V_1, V_2 and V_3. A negative T wave in V_5 and V_6 in the first week of life is not a sign of a pathological condition.

The QRS frontal axis is right deviated at +120°, which is normal in newborns.

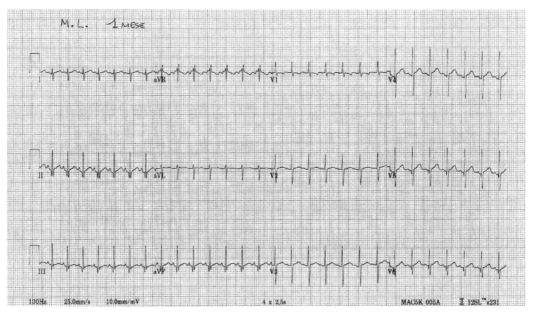

Fig. 1.22 Electrocardiogram recorded of a 27-day-old newborn

In Fig. 1.22, with regard to ventricular depolarization, a situation of balanced electrical forces in the ventricles can be seen; there is right ventricular dominance in V_1 and left ventricular dominance in V_6. Ventricular repolarization is normal since the T wave is negative in V_1 and positive in V_5 and V_6. This "infant pattern" can be present as early as the first few days of life. The QRS frontal axis is modestly right deviated at $+100°$, which is normal in the first month of life. This ECG is in accordance with the age of this patient, so it is normal.

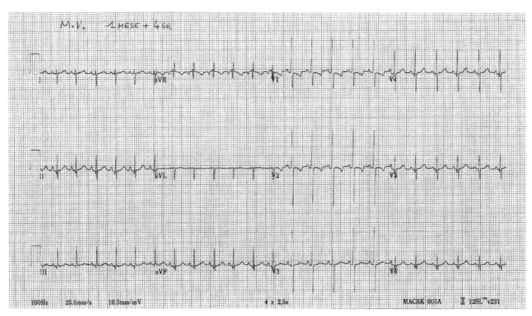

Fig. 1.23 Electrocardiogram recorded of a 35-day-old newborn

The observations made in Fig. 1.22 are also valid in this electrocardiogram sample (Fig. 1.23). The QRS axis here is more strongly right deviated at +120°, but is still within the normal range defined in this manual.

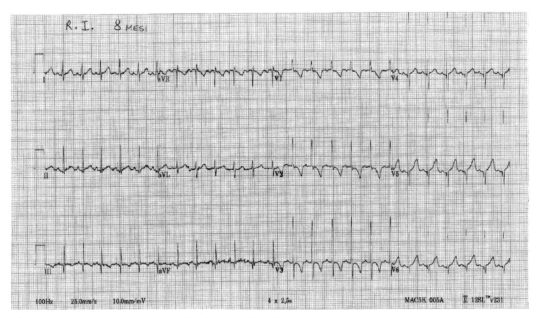

Fig. 1.24 Electrocardiogram recorded of an 8-month-old infant

This electrocardiogram sample (Fig. 1.24) shows a variant of the "infant pattern" of balanced electrical forces in the ventricles. Here, the R wave is exclusive in V_1 (the S wave of depolarizing electrical activity in the left ventricle is not represented). In order to judge this ECG as normal, the voltage of the R wave must be less than 1 mV. This is the case in this sample since the exclusive R wave has a voltage of 0.5 mV.

In V_6, the R wave, which represents left ventricular depolarization, dominates over the small S wave of right ventricular electrical forces. Ventricular repolarization is within the norm since the T wave is negative in V_1, V_2 and V_3, and positive in V_5 and V_6. The QRS frontal axis is normal at +65°.

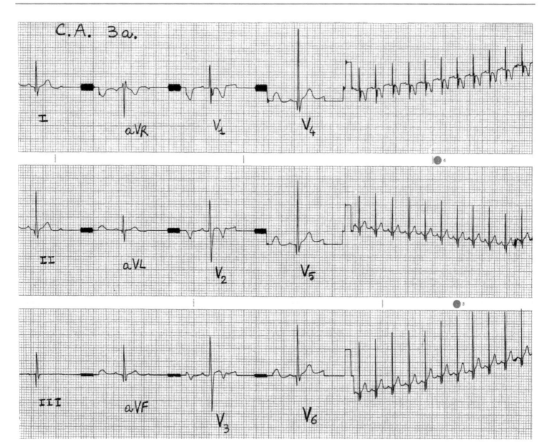

Fig. 1.25 Electrocardiogram recorded of a 3-year-old child

In Fig. 1.25, for V_1, the electrical forces of the right ventricle are prevalent such that R/S > 1. In V_6, however, the electrical forces of the left ventricle are prevalent, with a small S wave and a relationship of R/S > 1. This sets up a picture of balanced electrical forces in the ventricles that fits the "infant pattern", which can last up to the age of 3. Here, the age of the patient is in accordance with this electrocardiogram and thus, this trace should be considered normal.

The morphology of ventricular repolarization (with the T wave negative in V_1, V_2 and V_3, and positive in V_5 and V_6), and the QRS axis at +60°, help to define this ECG as normal.

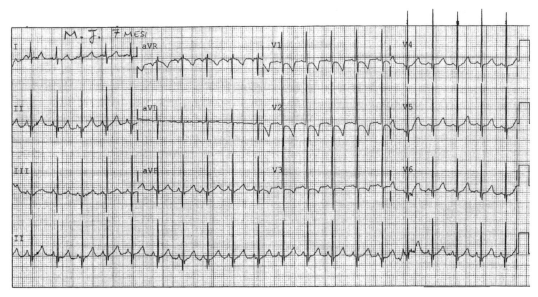

Fig. 1.26 Electrocardiogram recorded of a 7-month-old infant

In Fig. 1.26, with regard to ventricular depolarization, one can see balanced electrical forces in the ventricles. This is represented by electrical dominance of the right ventricle in V_1, in that R/S > 1, and electrical dominance of the left ventricle in V_6. This "infant pattern" is in accordance with the age of the patient and thus, is normal.

The situation with the ventricular repolarization is normal, with the T wave negative in V_1, V_2 and V_3 and positive in V_5 and V_6. At +80°, the QRS frontal axis is also within the normal range. Together these elements define this ECG as normal.

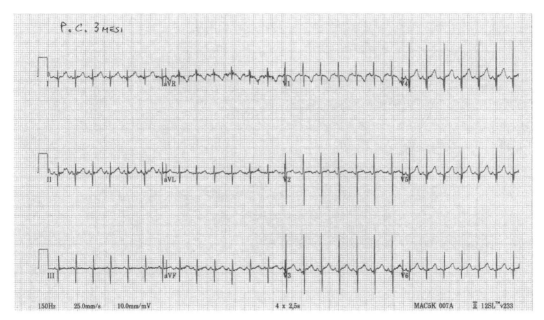

P. C. 3 MESI

Fig. 1.27 Electrocardiogram recorded of a 3-month-old infant

In Fig. 1.27, with regard to ventricular depolarization, we find balanced ventricular electrical forces in the precordial leads. In V_1, the electrical prevalence of the right ventricle is visible, with the R wave > the S wave such that R/S > 1. In V_6, the electrical forces of the left ventricle prevail with an absent S wave of right ventricular depolarization. The ECG therefore has the characteristics of the "infant pattern" with the variation of a deep Q wave in II, III and aV_F extremity leads with a voltage of 0.7 mV that is within the 1 mV limit defined by the norm.

In the electrical activity of ventricular repolarization, one can see that the T wave is negative in V_1 and positive in V_5 and V_6. The QRS frontal axis is within the norm at +90°. This electrocardiogram fits the "infant pattern", which is congruent with the age of the patient, thus this trace is normal.

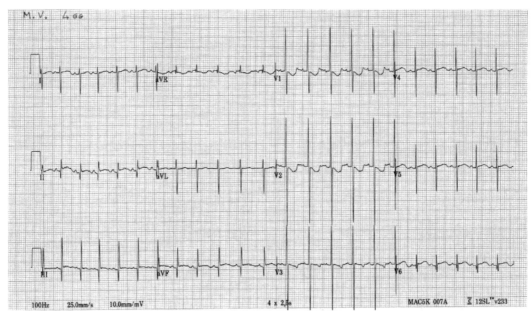

Fig. 1.28 Electrocardiogram recorded of a 4-day-old newborn

In the morphology of the precordial leads (Fig. 1.28), one can see the electrical activity of ventricular depolarization has balanced electrical forces in the ventricles. This is in line with the "infant pattern". As a variant, this can be present as early as the first few days of life. In V_1, one can see that the R wave of right ventricular depolarization has a voltage of 2.2 mV, which is at the upper limits of the norm, such that R/S > 1. In V_6, the R wave of left ventricular depolarization dominates, such that R/S > 1. The S wave of right ventricular depolarization has a voltage of 0.3 mV, which is within the 1 mV normal limit.

The electrical activity of ventricular repolarization is within the norm with the T wave negative in V_1, V_2 and V_3, and positive in V_5 and V_6. The QRS frontal axis is right deviated at +140°. This is within the norm for the first month of life. This trace can, therefore, be read as normal.

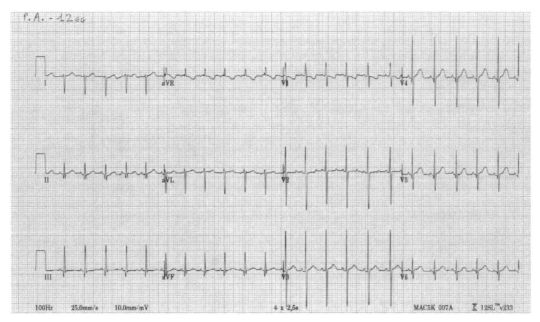

Fig. 1.29 Electrocardiogram recorded of a 12-day-old newborn

Considering the ventricular depolarization in Fig. 1.29, one can see balanced electrical forces in the ventricles, as in the previous ECG. This is represented by electrical dominance of the right ventricle in V_1 and electrical dominance of the left ventricle in V_6. As a variant of the norm, this "infant pattern" can already be present at a few days after birth.

Ventricular repolarization is normal since the T wave is negative in V_1, diphasic in V_2 and positive in V_5 and V_6. The QRS frontal axis is right deviated at +130°, which is normal in the first month of life. This ECG is therefore considered to be normal.

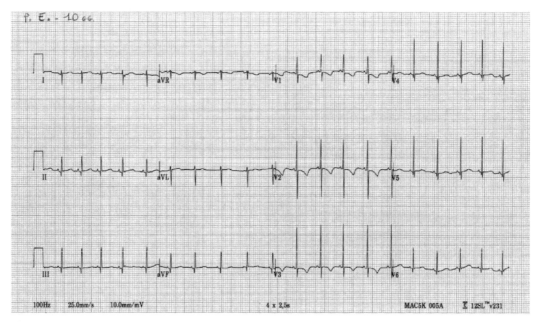

Fig. 1.30 Electrocardiogram recorded of a 10-day-old newborn

In Fig. 1.30, for V_1, the R wave (electrical forces of the right ventricle) dominates over the S wave (electrical forces of the left ventricle). In V_6, the R wave (electrical forces of the left ventricle) dominates. These elements indicate that the right and left ventricular electrical forces are balanced, meaning that this is the "infant pattern". As a variant of the norm, it can already be found in the first month of life. Ventricular repolarization is as it should be since the T wave is negative in V_1, V_2 and V_3; positive in V_5 and V_6. The QRS frontal axis is right deviated at +110°, which is normal for newborns. Together these elements define this trace as normal.

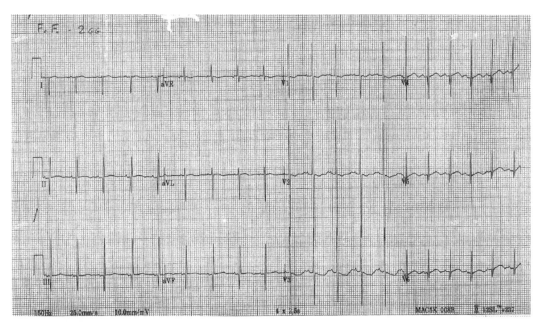

Fig. 1.31 Electrocardiogram recorded of a 2-day-old newborn

Considering the ventricular depolarization in Fig. 1.31, we see balanced electrical ventricular forces in the precordial leads. In V_1, the electrical forces of the right ventricle are prevalent with the R wave > S wave such that R/S > 1. Meanwhile in V_6, the electrical forces of the left ventricle prevail such that R/S > 1. Therefore, this fits the "infant pattern" that can already be present at birth as a variant of the norm. The deep 0.8 mV voltage Q wave in the II, III and aVF leads is within the 1 mV normal limit.

Regarding the electrical activity of ventricular repolarization, the flat/diphasic T wave in V_1–V_2 is also a variant of the norm in the first week of life. The parameters interpretated (sinus rhythm, a PR interval of 100 ms, QRS duration of 50 ms, QRS frontal axis of +130°, QTc interval of 428 ms) are in line with the normal ranges defined in this manual.

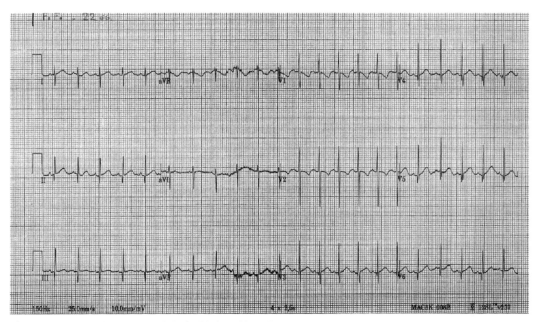

Fig. 1.32 Electrocardiogram recorded of a 22-day-old newborn

This ECG (Fig. 1.32) was recorded 20 days later on the same newborn as in Fig. 1.31. It is an example of the evolving morphology of the ECG pattern in the first few months of life.

With regard to the morphology of the V_1 and V_6 precordial leads, this trace still fits the "infant pattern" characteristics of the electrical activity of ventricular depolarization. In V_1–V_2, the T wave goes from flat to negative, as is normal after the first week of life, signifying the normal maturation of the pulmonary vascular bed, with a gradual fall in PVR.

In accordance with the gradual hemodynamic changes after birth, the reduction of right deviation of the QRS frontal axis (at +110°) indicates a growth of the "electrical mass" of the left ventricle at the expense of the right ventricle.

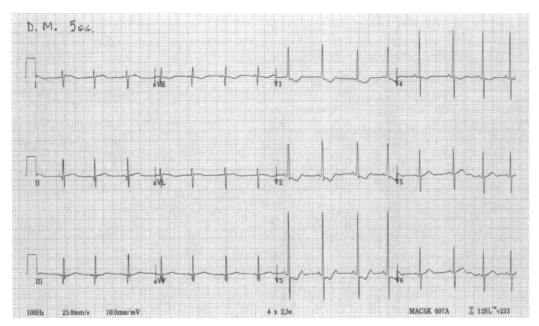

D. M. 5ᴳᴳ.

100Hz   25.0mm/s   10.0mm/mV   4 x 2,5s   MAC5K 007A   Σ 12SL™v233

Fig. 1.33 Electrocardiogram recorded of a 5-day-old newborn

Regarding the precordial leads in Fig. 1.33, the electrical forces in the ventricles are balanced, so this fits the "infant pattern", which is normal even for the first week of life. The uniqueness of the electrical dominance of the right ventricle in V_1 is shown here by a high voltage R wave of 15 mm (1.5 mV). It cannot be considered exclusive due to the presence of a miniscule S wave (0.1 mV) of left ventricular depolarization. In V_6, the left ventricle dominates such that R/S > 1. The morphology of ventricular repolarization is within the norm since the T wave is negative in V_1, V_2 and V_3 and positive in V_5 and V_6. The QRS frontal axis is right deviated at +110°, which is normal for a newborn.

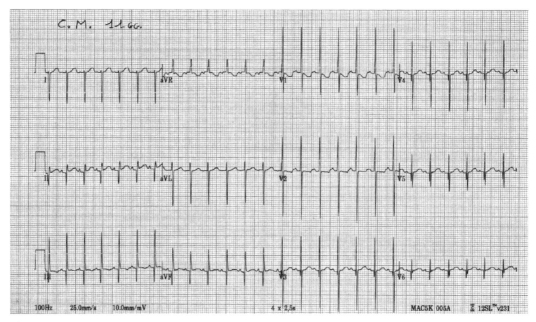

Fig. 1.34 Electrocardiogram recorded of an 11-day-old newborn

Regarding ventricular depolarization, the electrical forces in the ventricles are balanced in this trace (Fig. 1.34), as well. In V_1, the electrical forces of the right ventricle dominate. The R wave of right ventricular depolarization has a voltage of 2.2 mV, at the upper limits of the norm, and an S wave of left ventricular depolarization has a voltage of 1.1mV, such that R/S > 1. The electrical forces of the left ventricle dominate in V_6, such that R/S > 1. The deep Q wave in II, III and aV_F extremity leads has a voltage of 0.7 mV, which is within the normal limit of 1 mV, and therefore is normal.

Ventricular repolarization is normal since the T wave is negative in V_1, diphasic in V_2 and positive in V_5 and V_6. The QRS frontal axis shows right deviation at +160°, which is within the norm for a newborn during the first month of life. As a variant of the norm, this "infant pattern" can already be present in the first few days of life.

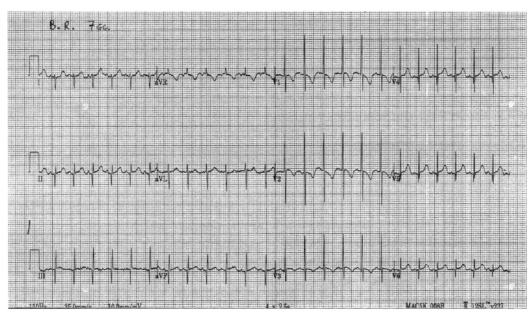

Fig. 1.35 Electrocardiogram recorded of a 7-day-old newborn

In Fig. 1.35, when considering the precordial leads, the electrical forces of the ventricles are balanced. V_1 shows right dominance since the R wave of right ventricular depolarization has a voltage at the upper limits of the norm (2 mV) and the S wave of left ventricular depolarization is well represented at 0.9 mV such that R/S > 1. V_6 shows left dominance with an R wave of 0.5 mV, but no S wave of right ventricular depolarization. The deep, 0.7 mV Q wave in II, III and aV_F extremity leads does not surpass the 1 mV normal limit and so is considered normal.

Ventricular repolarization is normal since the T wave is negative in V_1, V_2 and V_3, and positive in V_5 and V_6. The QRS frontal axis shows right deviation at +150°, which is normal for newborns (in the first month of life). As a variant of the norm, the "infant pattern" can already be present in the first few days of life.

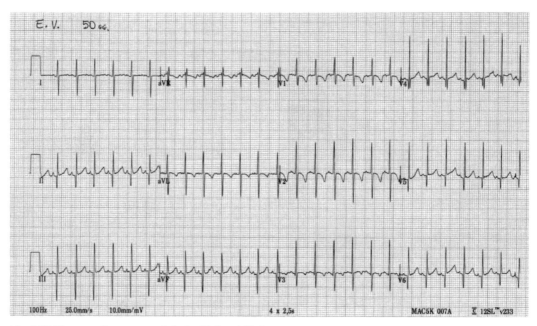

Fig. 1.36 Electrocardiogram recorded of a 50-day-old infant

With regard to the precordial leads (Fig. 1.36), the electrical forces of the ventricles are balanced. In V_1, the R wave of right ventricular depolarization dominates over the S wave of left ventricular depolarization such that R/S > 1. In V_6, the electrical activity of the left ventricle dominates such that there is no S wave of right ventricular depolarization. In this case, the "infant pattern" shows a deep Q wave, which is at the upper limit of the norm for amplitude (10 mm, or 1 mV) in II, III, aV_F and V_6 leads, and is considered a variant of the norm.

The morphology of ventricular repolarization is normal since the T wave is negative in V_1–V_2–V_3 and positive in V_5–V_6. The QRS frontal axis is normal at +95°. This trace shows the "infant pattern", which is congruent with the age of the patient and thus, is normal.

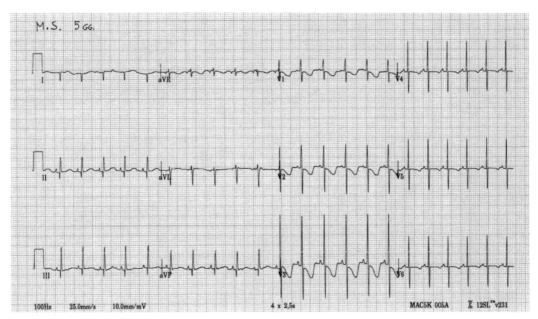

M.S. 5 GG.

100Hz   25.0mm/s   10.0mm/mV   4 x 2,5s   MAC5K 005A   ⅀ 12SL™v231

Fig. 1.37 Electrocardiogram recorded of a 5-day-old newborn

For ventricular depolarization, this trace (Fig. 1.37) also presents balanced electrical forces in the ventricles. This is evident in the electrical dominance of the right ventricle in V_1, such that R/S > 1, and the electrical dominance of the left ventricle in V_6, such that R/S > 1. As a variant of the norm, this "infant pattern" can already be present in the first few days of life.

The morphology of ventricular repolarization is normal since the T wave is negative in V_1, V_2 and V_3, and flat/negative in V_5 and V_6. This is a variant of the norm during the first week of life. The QRS frontal axis is right deviated at +120°, which is normal in the first month of life. These elements define this ECG as normal.

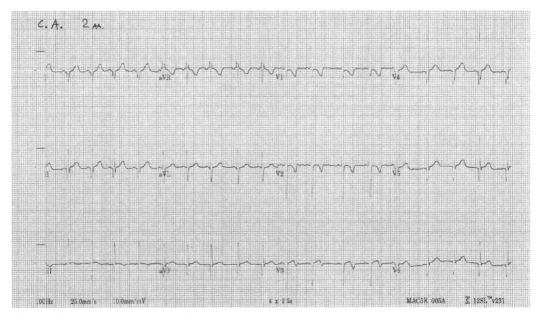

Fig. 1.38 Electrocardiogram recorded of a 2-year-old child

In Fig. 1.38, for V_1, the electrical forces of the right ventricle are prevalent such that R/S > 1. In V_6, the electrical forces of the left ventricle are prevalent and the S wave is very small such that R/S > 1. V_1 and V_6 make up a picture of balanced electrical forces, fitting the "infant pattern", which can last up to the age of 3. In this case, the age of the patient is in accordance with the electrocardiographic pattern, so the ECG is to be considered normal.

The morphology of ventricular repolarization (with the T wave negative in V_1–V_2–V_3, and positive in V_5–V_6) and the QRS frontal axis at +50° also contribute to defining this electrocardiogram as normal.

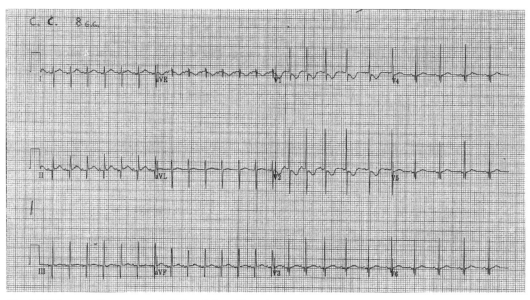

Fig. 1.39 Electrocardiogram recorded of an 8-day-old newborn

Regarding the precordial leads, the electrical forces, in Fig. 1.39, of the ventricles are visibly balanced. In V_1, the electrical forces of the right ventricle are dominant such that R/S > 1. In V_6, the electrical forces of the left ventricle are dominant such that R/S > 1. The deep, 0.5 mV Q wave in II, III, and aV_F leads is within the normal limit of 1 mV and so, is to be considered a variant of the norm.

Ventricular repolarization is normal since the T wave is negative in V_1 and V_2, and positive in V_5 and V_6. The QRS frontal axis is right deviated at +120°, which is normal for newborns (the first month of life). As a variant of the norm, the "infant pattern" can already be present in the first few days of life, therefore this ECG is to be read as normal.

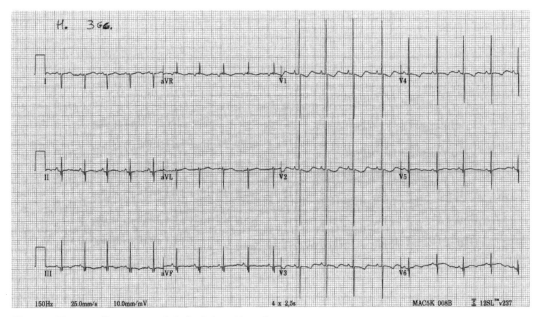

Fig. 1.40 Electrocardiogram recorded of a 3-day-old newborn

The electrical forces of the ventricles are visibly balanced in Fig. 1.40 as well, since R/S > 1 in V_1 and R/S > 1 in V_6. This is in accordance with the "infant pattern" which can already be present in the first few days of life as a variation of the norm.

In relation to the age of the patient (first week of life), the morphology of ventricular repolarization and the +135° right deviated QRS frontal axis fit the normal standards. The T wave is diphasic in V_1 and V_2, negative in V_3 and V_4, and positive in V_5 and V_6. This trace is therefore considered to be normal.

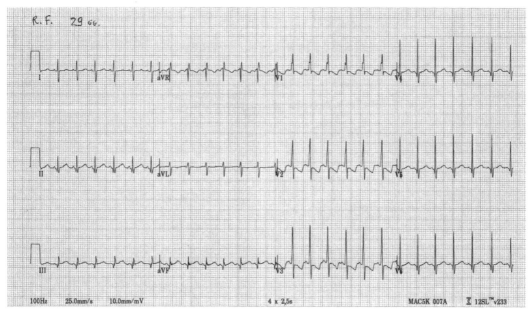

Fig. 1.41 Electrocardiogram recorded of a 29-day-old newborn

In Fig. 1.41, the electrical forces of ventricular depolarization are balanced such that R/S > 1 in V_1 and R/S > 1 in V_6. This "infant pattern" trace shows slightly delayed right intraventricular conduction, which is evident in V_1 through the slurring in the rise of the R wave, and in V_6 through the morphology of the slightly widened S wave.

The morphology of ventricular repolarization (with the T wave negative in V_1, V_2 and V_3, and positive in V_5 and V_6) and the QRS frontal axis at +90° is normal. Over all, this ECG is appropriate for the age of the patient and therefore is normal.

1.3   The Adult Pattern

The adult pattern is characterized by prevalent electrical activity in the left ventricle. This ECG pattern is the norm after 2–3 years of life.

This last morphological change that the pediatric ECG goes through is as a direct consequence of hemodynamic and anatomic changes described earlier in this manual, which bring about the typical adult condition of the left ventricular predominance.

Since the electrical forces of the left ventricle dominate, in the V_1 lead the S wave will dominate over the R wave such that R/S < 1. The S wave in V_1 represents the depolarizing electrical activity of the left ventricle. To be considered normal, the voltage of the S wave must be less than 25 mm (2.5 mV). In the V_6 precordial lead, the R wave will dominate over the S wave such that R/S > 1. The R wave in V_6 represents the depolarizing electrical activity of the left ventricle. To be considered normal the voltage of the R wave must be less than 25 mm (2.5 mV) and the S wave (the depolarizing electrical activity of the right ventricle) must have a voltage less than 5 mm (0.5 mV). According to the requisites of the norm, there can never be an exclusive R wave in V_1 (see Table 1.5).

At times, even in the first month of a normal newborn's life, an ECG can show an adult pattern of dominant depolarizing electrical forces of the left ventricle. In these cases, the useful elements in judging a trace as normal are: the voltage of the S wave in V_1, the voltage of the R wave in V_4–V_5–V_6, the morphology of the T wave and the QRS frontal axis.

In terms of the repolarizing electrical activity of the ventricles (the morphology of the T wave), the "adult pattern" is characterized by a positive T wave in V_6 and a negative T wave in V_1–V_2–V_3 up until adolescence (in girls, even later) (Table 1.6). A positive T wave in V_2 and V_3 is, nonetheless, a variant of the norm.

Table 1.5 Adult pattern of ventricular depolarization. Left ventricular prevalence is the norm in the "adult pattern"

QRS – Adult pattern	
In V_1: S wave dominant such that R/S < 1	S wave < 25 mm
In V_6: R wave dominant such that R/S > 1	R wave < 25 mm, S wave < 5 mm
In V_1: R wave never exclusive	

Table 1.6 Adult pattern of ventricular repolarization

T wave – Adult pattern	
In V_1–V_2–V_3: negative	even up to adolescence
In V_6: positive	

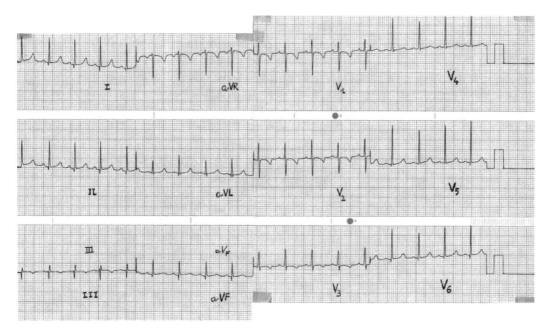

Fig. 1.42 Electrocardiogram recorded of a 3-year-old child

In Fig. 1.42, for V_1, the S wave (the electrical forces of the left ventricle) is dominant such that R/S < 1. In V_6, the R wave (again the electrical forces of the left ventricle) is dominant with no S wave of right ventricular depolarization. These elements make up a picture of left ventricular prevalence, which is the norm for the "adult pattern" of ventricular depolarization. The "adult pattern" is normal after the age of 2–3, so this trace is congruent with the age of the patient, thus making it normal.

Together the +30° QRS frontal axis and the morphology of ventricular repolarization (with the T wave negative in V_1, V_2 and V_3, and positive in V_5 and V_6) define this ECG as normal.

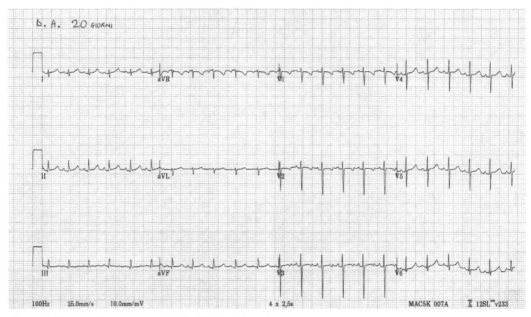

Fig. 1.43 Electrocardiogram recorded of a 20-day-old newborn

In this trace (Fig. 1.43), one can see the electrical dominance of the left ventricle. In V_1, the S wave is dominant, that is, the depolarizing electrical forces of the left ventricle are prevalent such that R/S < 1. In V_6, the R wave is dominant also meaning the depolarizing electrical forces of the left ventricle are prevalent such that R/S > 1. The voltage of the S wave in V_1 and the R wave in V_6 is normal. Ventricular repolarization is normal with the T wave negative in V_1–V_2 and positive in V_6. The QRS frontal axis is normal at +70°. As is sometimes the case, this "adult pattern" is already present in the first month of life in the absence of organic cardiopathy.

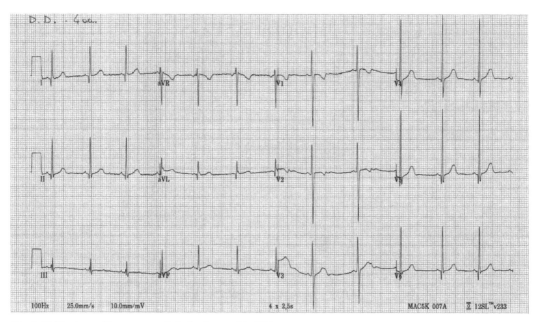

Fig. 1.44 Electrocardiogram recorded of a 4-year-old child

In Fig. 1.44, with regard to the morphology of ventricular depolarization, the electrical prevalence of the left ventricle is visible in the V_1 and V_6 precordial leads. This situation is characteristic of the "adult pattern" and is appropriate for the age of this patient.

Ventricular repolarization is normal with the T wave negative in V_1 and V_2, and positive in V_5 and V_6. The +50° QRS frontal axis is normal after the first year of life. All these elements identify this ECG as normal.

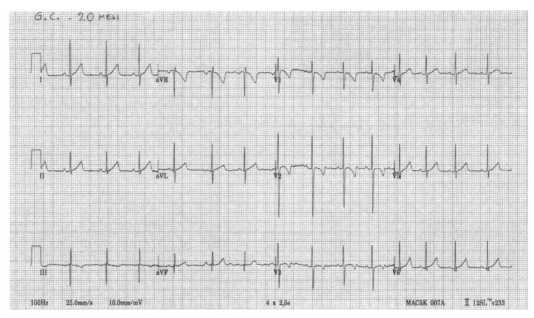

Fig. 1.45 Electrocardiogram recorded of a 20-month-old child

In V_1, the S wave, the electrical forces of the left ventricle, is dominant in that $R/S < 1$. In V_6, the R wave, which also refers to the electrical forces of the left ventricle, is dominant. These elements constitute a picture of left ventricular prevalence, which is standard in the "adult pattern" of ventricular depolarization. The "adult pattern" is normal after 2–3 years of age and is already present here at 20 months (Fig. 1.45).

Together, the +30° QRS axis and the morphology of ventricular repolarization (with the T wave negative in V_1, V_2 and V_3, and positive in V_5 and V_6) contribute to defining this ECG as normal.

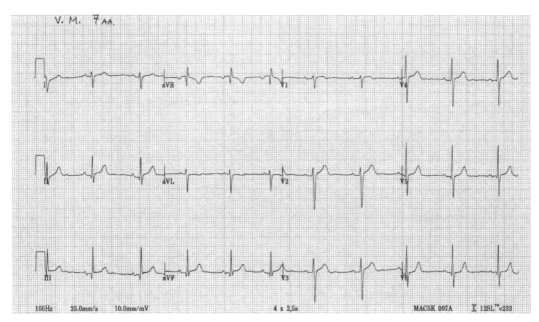

Fig. 1.46 Electrocardiogram recorded of a 7-year-old child

Since the left ventricle has electrical dominance, this trace (Fig. 1.46) fits the "adult pattern" of ventricular depolarization. There is a slight delay of right intraventricular conduction in the QRS morphology in V_1. This is confirmed by the morphology of the S wave in V_6. The still slightly right deviated QRS frontal axis (+110°) is a variant of the norm, as is ventricular repolarization, since the T wave is diphasic in V_1, and positive in V_2–V_3 and V_5–V_6.

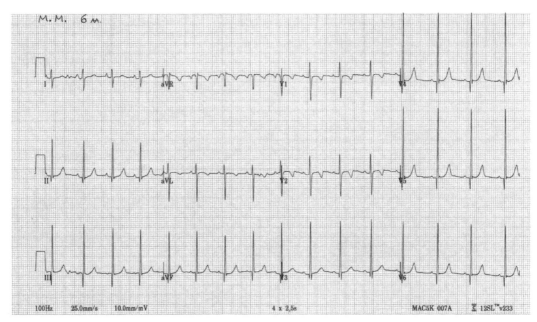

Fig. 1.47 Electrocardiogram recorded of a 6-year-old child

   In V_1, the S wave, the electrical force of the left ventricle, is dominant such that R/S < 1. In V_6, the R wave is dominant and the S wave of the right ventricular depolarization is absent (Fig. 1.47). This means that, once again, the electrical forces of the left ventricle are prevalent. These elements make up a picture of left ventricular prevalence, which is normal in the "adult pattern" of ventricular depolarization. This "adult pattern" trace is in accordance with the age of the patient since it is the norm after 2–3 years of age.
   The +95° QRS frontal axis is normal, as is the morphology of ventricular repolarization, since the T wave is negative in V_1 and V_2, and positive in V_5 and V_6.

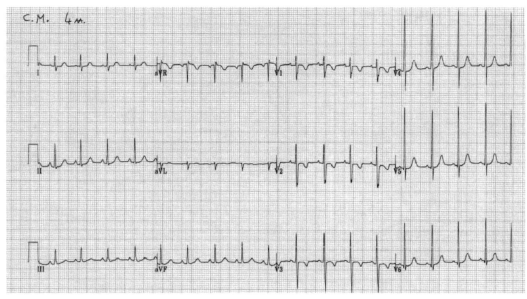

Fig. 1.48 Electrocardiogram recorded of a 4-year-old child

In Fig. 1.48, with regard to the precordial leads, in V_1, the S wave, the electrical forces of the left ventricle, is dominant such that R/S < 1, while in V_6, the R wave is dominant such that R/S > 1. This means that, once again the electrical forces of the left ventricle are prevalent. These elements make up a picture of left ventricular prevalence, which is normal in the "adult pattern" of ventricular depolarization, and is congruous for the age of the patient. The +60° QRS frontal axis and the morphology of ventricular repolarization (with the T wave negative in V_1, V_2 and V_3, and positive in V_5–V_6) also contribute to defining this ECG as normal.

Along with the heart rhythm evaluation, the following basic parameters are initially considered when reading an ECG:

- Heart rate
- PR interval
- QRS frontal axis
- QRS duration
- QT and QTc (heart rate corrected) interval.

In pediatric ECGs these parameters show different values from those of adults.

The normal range of adult **heart rate** is 60–100 beats/minute. A heart rate below this range is refered to as bradycardia and above this range, as tachycardia. Newborns and infants habitually show higher heart rate compared to adults. From birth through to the age of 1, the normal range is between 110 and 180 beats per minute, although transitory sinus bradycardia up to 80 beats per minute is a physiological phenomenon, particularly during sleep.

After the age of 1, the heart rate values gradually reduce, finally reaching those of an adult. Roughly, from age 1 to 6 the normal range is between 90 and 130 beats per minute and from age 6 to 12, between 60 and 110 beats per minute.

If a newborn or infant, at rest, has a persistent and stable heart rate over 180 beats per minute, it is prudent to record an ECG to exclude tachyarrhythmia.

The normal **duration** range of the adult **PR interval** is between 120 ms and 220 ms. PR interval duration below this range is called *short PR* and above it is called *first degree atrioventricular block*. In pediatrics, the PR interval is generally shorter, with upper limits of the norm varying in relation to age and heart rate.

As described in Table 2.1, the normal range in the first month of life is between 80 ms and 120 ms. Then from 2 months of age up to 1 year, it is between 80 ms and 140 ms. From the age of 1 to 5, it is between 100 ms and 160 ms and from the age of 6 to 12, it is between 110 ms and 180 ms.

The normal adult **QRS duration** is 100 ms at the highest. Over that is considered a complete right or left bundle branch block. In pediatrics, the QRS duration is shorter because the size of the heart is smaller, and consequently, so are the electrical circuits and the myocardial mass. The period of ventricular depolarization is thus shorter.

In the first month of life the upper limit of the norm of the QRS duration is 65 ms. From infancy (the second month of life), up to the age of 8 the upper limit of the norm is considered 80 ms. After the age of 8, the upper limit of the norm is the same as that of adults (see Table 2.2).

M. A. Galli (✉)
Perinatal and Pediatric Cardiology
Ospedale Maggiore Policlinico
Milan, Italy
e-mail: mariellagalli@gmail.com

M. A. Galli, G. B. Danzi, *A Guide to Neonatal and Pediatric ECGs*,
DOI: 10.1007/978-88-470-2856-2_2, © Springer-Verlag Italia 2013

Table 2.1 Duration of PR interval (in milliseconds). Normal ranges

Age range	PR interval range
In the first month of life	80 ms–120 ms
From 2 months to age 1	80 ms–140 ms
From age 1 to 5	100 ms–160 ms
From age 6 to 12	110 ms–180 ms

Table 2.2 QRS duration (in milliseconds)

Age range	QRS duration
In the 1st month of life	< 65 ms
From infancy to age 8	< 80 ms
From age 8–16	< 100 ms

The **QT interval** is an important parameter in pediatric ECGs because its increase is an indicator of cardiac electrical instability, and thus of arrhythmia risk. Measured in milliseconds, the QT interval encompasses the beginning of the QRS complex and the end of the T wave. It corresponds to the depolarization and repolarization of the common myocardium. It is generally measured in the II extremity lead and in the V_5 and V_6 precordial leads, considering the longest value. The QT interval is dependent on heart rate and is corrected by using Bazett's formula. Therefore, this involves the corrected QT interval (QTc) whose normal value is less than 440 ms in children and adult males, while in women the upper limit of the norm is 470 ms. Bazett's formula is: QTc = QT (ms)/square root of RR, where RR is the time interval in ms between two successive R waves.

The **QRS frontal axis** expresses the orientation of electrical ventricular forces. This means it gives an indication of the work and weight of the ventricles. By making reference to the Cabrera circle, it allows one to establish if ventricular depolarization occurs on the whole with a general normal direction; if it is directed to the left when the electrical mass of

the left ventricle is prevalent; or if it is directed to the right when the electrical mass of the right ventricle is prevalent.

The normal range of the QRS frontal axis in adults is from 0° to 90° (+60° is the 50th percentile). The reason for this is that when the electrical ratio between the two ventricles is normal, the left ventricle is dominant in terms of electrical force because it pumps against the high resistance of the peripheral vascular bed, and so has a myocardial mass and an electrical mass that are higher than the right ventricle, which pumps against the low resistance of the pulmonary vascular bed. In children, particularly in the first month of life, the right ventricle has greater electrical mass than the left due to the fetal hemodynamic condition. After the 31st week of gestation, the right ventricle, which pumps against the high resistance of the pulmonary vascular bed, develops a higher myocardial mass and electrical mass than the left ventricle, which pumps against the low resistance of the placental vascular bed. For newborns, the normal QRS frontal axis is over +120° right deviated and in the first week of life this can be strained (+180°/+210°).

Over the next several months, (allowing for individual variation) the normal process of

Table 2.3 QRS frontal axis (in degrees)

Age range	QRS frontal axis
In the 1st month of life	over +120° (right deviated) up to +180°/+210° in the 1st week of life
After the 6th month of life	under +120°
After the age of 1	under +100°

remodeling or maturation of the pulmonary vascular bed brings about the gradual reduction of pulmonary vascular resistance (PVR). This in turn brings about a reduction in the myocardial mass and electrical force of the right ventricle. In contrast, the left ventricle, which pumps against the high resistance of the peripheral vascular bed after birth, slowly gains myocardial mass and electrical force. Thus, the QRS frontal axis progressively reduces its right deviation and turns toward the left. Except for individual variation, the QRS frontal axis generally comes in under +120° after 6 months of life, and under +100° after the age of 1 (see Table 2.3).

While the left and superior frontal QRS axis in adults is defined as at least a -30° QRS axis, during the first month of life, it is defined as less than +30°.

In children, the QRS frontal axis directed to the left should be regarded with suspicion because it is a typical marker of some congenital heart diseases: complete form of atrioventricular septal defect or atrioventricular canal defect, ostium primum atrial septal defect, *inlet-type* ventricular septal defect, atrioventricular septal defect with tetralogy of Fallot, tricuspid atresia, Ebstein's anomaly of the tricuspid valve, and univentricular heart with double inlet.

The leftward and superior QRS frontal axis can be present even in pediatric patients with structurally normal hearts, as a sign of a simple delay in intraventricular conduction (anterior fascicular block). These normal structures, however, should always be prudently confirmed by a physical examination and in case of doubt, an echocardiogram.

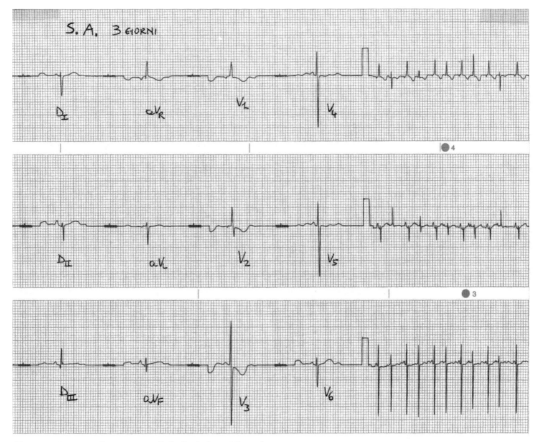

Fig. 2.1 Electrocardiogram recorded of a 3-day-old newborn

This trace (Fig. 2.1) is an example of a very pronounced right deviated QRS frontal axis (about +180°), which is a variation of the norm in the first week of life.

Regarding the V_1 and V_6 precordial leads, the "neonatal pattern" is immediately recognizable. The prevalent electrical force of the right ventricle is congruous with the age of the patient, and thus, normal. The morphology of ventricular repolarization is normal since the T wave is negative in V_1, V_2 and V_3, and positive in V_5 and V_6.

D. M. 5 GG.
I
aVR
V1
V4
II
aVL
V2
V5
III
aVF
V3
V6
150Hz
25.0mm/s
10.0mm/mV
4 x 2.5s
MAC5K 008B
12SL™v237

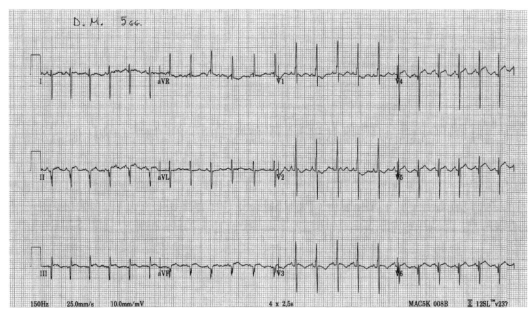

Fig. 2.2 Electrocardiogram recorded of a 5-day-old newborn

In this example (Fig. 2.2), the right axial deviation is extreme (+210°) and the QRS is totally positive on aV_R, which is a variant of the norm in the first week of life.

The electrical forces of the right ventricle are dominant in V_1 and V_6, so this is the "neonatal pattern" of ventricular depolarization. This ECG is normal considering the age of the patient. The pattern of ventricular repolarization is also normal since the T wave is diphasic in V_1–V_2 and positive in V_5–V_6.

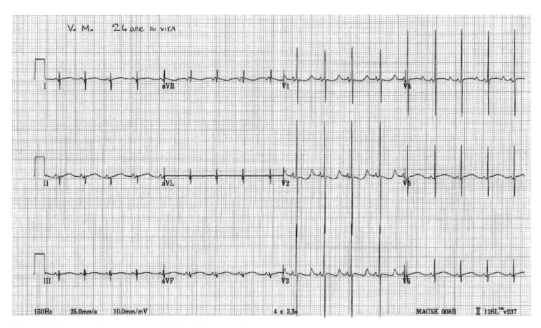

Fig. 2.3 Electrocardiogram recorded of a 24-hour-old newborn

In this trace (Fig. 2.3), the QRS frontal axis shows right deviation at +180°, which is a variation of the norm during the first week of life. The electrical forces of the ventricles are balanced. In V_1, the right ventricle is dominant and in V_6 the left ventricle is dominant, so this is the "infant pattern" of ventricular depolarization. As a variation of the norm, this morphology can already be present at birth.

Ventricular repolarization is normal since the T wave is diphasic in V_1–V_2–V_3 and positive in V_5–V_6. The aspects analyzed in this ECG are considered normal in relation to the patient's age.

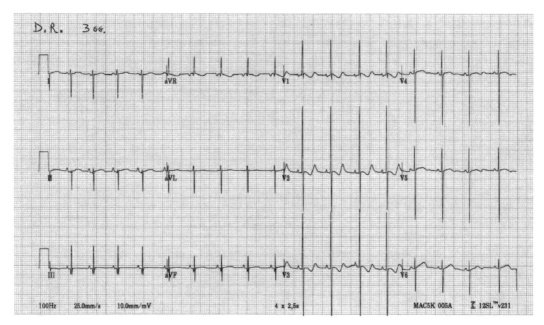

Fig. 2.4 Electrocardiogram recorded of a 3-day-old newborn

In this case (Fig. 2.4), the QRS frontal axis shows strain and right deviation (about +190°), which is a variant of the norm in the first week of life.

The electrical depolarization of the ventricles fits the "neonatal pattern" since the right ventricle is dominant in V_1 and V_6. The morphology of ventricular repolarization is normal since the T wave is diphasic in V_1, V_2 and V_3, and positive in V_6. These elements are congruous with the age of the patient. Together, these elements define this ECG as normal.

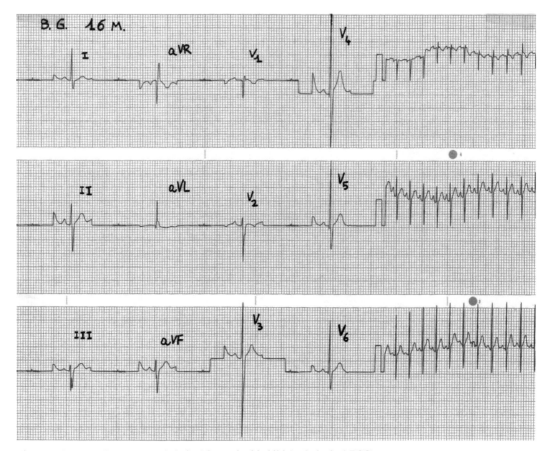

Fig. 2.5 Electrocardiogram recorded of a 16-month-old child (pathological ECG)

In this trace (Fig. 2.5), the pathological element is the QRS frontal axis directed to the left (-30°). There is a slight delay in right intraventricular conduction. The morphology of ventricular repolarization is normal. The patient suffered from a complete form of atrioventricular septal defect, which was surgically corrected.

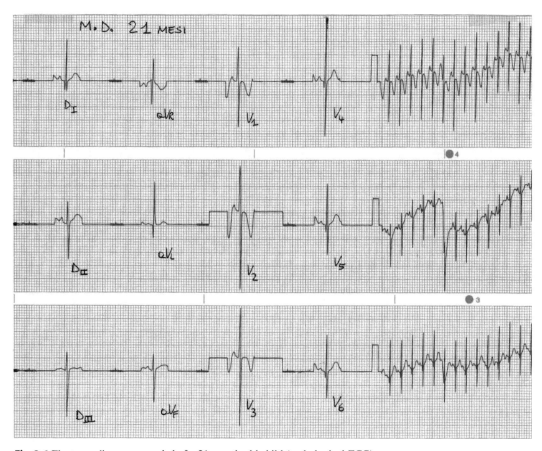

Fig. 2.6 Electrocardiogram recorded of a 21-month-old child (pathological ECG)

This is an example of a pathological leftward and superior frontal QRS axis (-30°) (Fig. 2.6). Otherwise this ECG is within normal limits. The patient suffered from ostium primum atrial septal defect.

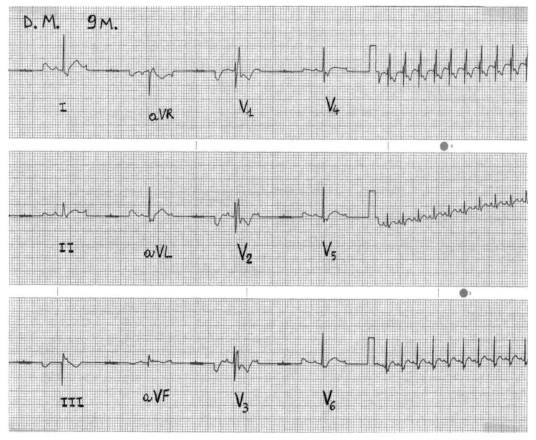

Fig. 2.7 Electrocardiogram recorded of a 9-month-old infant (pathological ECG)

In this trace (Fig. 2.7), the pathological elements are a leftward and superior frontal QRS axis (-30°) and a right bundle branch block (the QRS duration is about 100 ms, which is above the 80 ms limit for infants). The patient suffered from Ebstein's anomaly of the tricuspid valve.

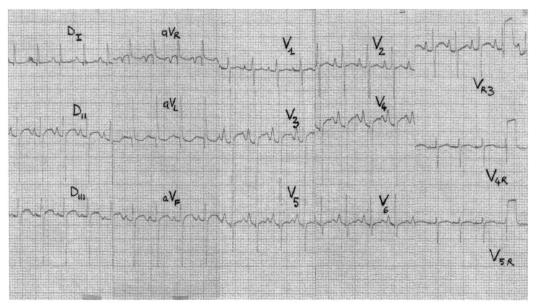

Fig. 2.8 Electrocardiogram recorded of a 35-day-old infant (pathological ECG)

In this trace (Fig. 2.8), the pathological elements are, essentially, the leftward and superior frontal QRS axis (-30°), the electrical prevalence of the left ventricle in V_1 and in V_6, and the morphology of ventricular repolarization. Specifically, the T wave is positive in V_1–V_2, indicating right ventricular systolic load and negative in aV_L with the appearance of left ventricular overload.

This chart should be read as pathological due to the signs of biventricular overload. The patient suffered from a complete form of atrioventricular septal defect.

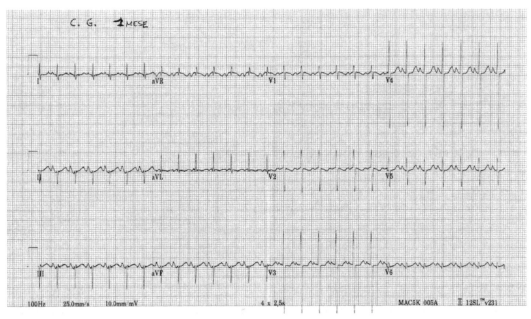

Fig. 2.9 Electrocardiogram recorded of a 32-day-old infant (pathological ECG)

In Fig. 2.9, the QRS frontal axis is pathologically left deviated at -60°. This pattern of ventricular depolarization fits the "infant pattern", which is appropriate for the age of the patient and thus, normal. The patient suffered from tricuspid atresia.

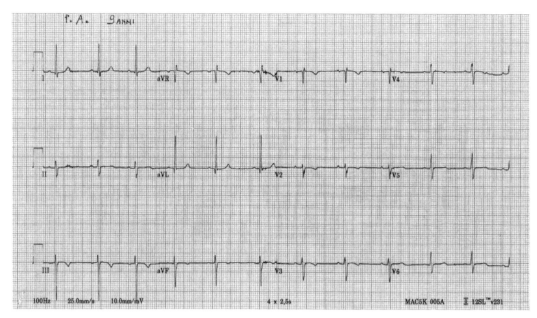

Fig. 2.10 Electrocardiogram recorded of a 9-year-old child (pathological ECG)

In this trace (Fig. 2.10), the pathological element is the leftward and superior frontal QRS axis (-40°). A slight delay in right intraventricular conduction is also visible. The morphology of ventricular repolarization is normal. This patient suffered from a form of atrioventricular septal defect, which was surgically corrected.

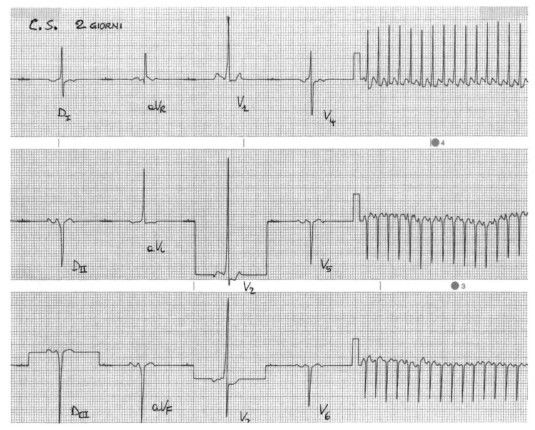

Fig. 2.11 Electrocardiogram recorded of a 2-day-old newborn (pathological ECG)

Two pathological elements are visible in this trace (Fig. 2.11): the pronounced left axis deviation (-70°) and a short PR interval (60 ms). The latter is associated with a slur on the upstroke of the QRS (delta wave of ventricular pre-excitation), which is evident especially in V_1–V_2–V_3 and I–aV_L leads. The patient suffered from ventricular pre-excitation.

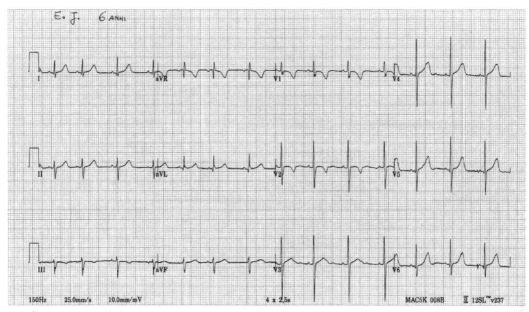

Fig. 2.12 Electrocardiogram recorded of a 6-year-old child

The QRS frontal axis directed to the left (-40°) is the only visible anomaly in this trace (Fig. 2.12); in fact, the morphology of ventricular depolarization and repolarization is normal.

An echocardiographic evaluation uncovered no alterations in cardiac structure and in this case, the QRS frontal axis directed to the left showed a simple delay in intraventricular conduction (anterior fascicular block).

Part II
Pathological Scenarios

Right Ventricular Overload

3.1 Right Ventricular Systolic Overload

Right ventricular systolic overload refers to an overload of systolic pressure in the right ventricle and it indicates a right ventricle that pumps more than the normal 30 mmHg while developing systolic pressure. This hemodynamic situation appears in the following conditions:

1. All congenital heart defects that obstruct right ventricular outflow, i.e. significant or critical pulmonary valve stenosis, pulmonary atresia, and Tetralogy of Fallot
2. Congenital heart defects causing pulmonary hypertension from a high pulmonary blood flow with low pulmonary vascular resistance, for example a large ventricular septal defect, double-outlet right ventricle, complete form of atrioventricular septal defect, total anomalous pulmonary venous drainage
3. Congenital heart defects complicated by pulmonary artery hypertension due to progressive structural abnormalities in the

pulmonary vascular bed, i.e. obstructive pulmonary vascular disease.

In electrocardiograms, right ventricular systolic overload is expressed as right ventricular hypertrophy, which is a persistence of the "neonatal pattern" of right ventricular prevalence after the first month of life.

In terms of the V_1 and V_6 precordial leads, the ECG pattern shows that the electrical forces of the right ventricle are prevalent. In V_1, the R wave of right ventricular depolarization will dominate over the S wave of left ventricular depolarization in that R/S > 1 and the R wave > 20 mm (> 2 mV). Alternatively, the R wave can be exclusive with a voltage over 10 mm (> 1 mV), or a qR aspect; any Q wave in the V_1 lead usually results from severe pressure or volume load of the right ventricle. In V_6, the S wave of the right ventricular depolarization will dominate over the R wave of left ventricular depolarization such that R/S < 1. Alternatively, when R/S > 1, the S wave > 10 mm (> 1 mV).

Regarding the electrical activity of ventricular repolarization, it is necessary to look at the morphology of the T wave in V_1 and V_2. An upright T wave after the first week of life generally signifies right ventricular systolic load.

These elements can also be accompanied by a pathological right deviation of the QRS frontal axis, which is inappropriate for the age of the patient (see Table 3.1).

M. A. Galli (✉)
Perinatal and Pediatric Cardiology
Ospedale Maggiore Policlinico
Milan, Italy
e-mail: mariellagalli@gmail.com

M. A. Galli, G. B. Danzi, *A Guide to Neonatal and Pediatric ECGs*,
DOI: 10.1007/978-88-470-2856-2_3, © Springer-Verlag Italia 2013

Table 3.1 Right ventricular systolic overload or pressure overload. Right ventricular hypertrophy electrocardiographically defined by the persistence of the "neonatal pattern" of right ventricular prevalence after the first month of life

In V_1	Exclusive R wave > 10 mm
	R/S > 1 with R wave > 20 mm
	qR aspect
In V_6	R/S < 1
	R/S > 1 with S wave > 10 mm
In V_1	Positive T wave after the 1st week of life

Pathological right deviation of the QRS frontal axis (inappropriate for age)

It is worth repeating that it is crucial to refer to the age of the patient when judging an electrocardiographical anomaly and making a diagnosis of right ventricular hypertrophy. The "neonatal pattern" should be confined to the first month of life, after which, it is incongruous with the age of the patient and right ventricular prevalence becomes a sign of right ventricular hypertrophy.

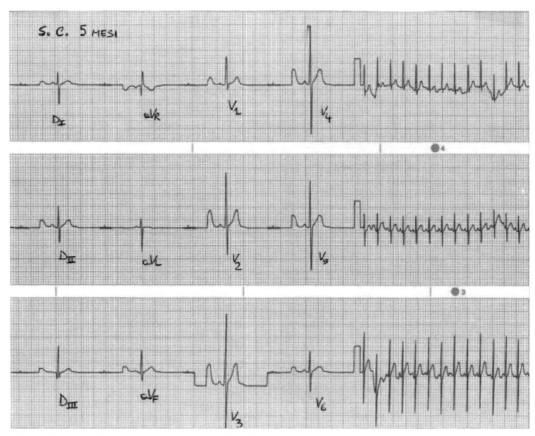

Fig. 3.1 Electrocardiogram recorded of a 5-month-old infant

   In this trace (Fig. 3.1), the sign of right ventricular hypertrophy is the appearance of right ventricular electrical prevalence in V_1 and V_6. This fits the "neonatal pattern" which is incongruous with the age of the patient. In V_1, the right ventricle is electrically dominant with the R wave > the S wave such that R/S > 1. The same is true in V_6 where the amplitude of the S wave of right ventricular depolarization is equal to that of the R wave such that R/S = 1.

   The electrical activity of ventricular repolarization indicates right ventricular systolic overload since the T wave is positive in V_1–V_2. The QRS axis is right deviated at about +130°. Therefore, this ECG is pathological due to signs of right ventricular hypertrophy. The patient suffered from congenital pulmonary valve stenosis.

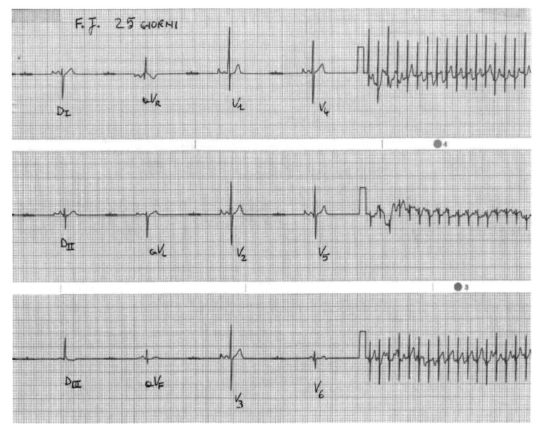

Fig. 3.2 Electrocardiogram recorded of a 25-day-old newborn

In this case (Fig. 3.2), the "neonatal pattern" of electrical prevalence of the right ventricle is recognizable in V_1 (R wave > S wave, such that R/S > 1) and in V_6 (S wave > R wave, such that R/S < 1) and is congruous with the age of this 25-day-old patient. The +160° right deviation of the QRS axis is within the norm during the first month of life. The upright T wave in V_1–V_2 is the only sign that indicates a pathological condition, in this case, right ventricular systolic load. In fact, the patient suffered from slight congenital pulmonary valve stenosis.

M.E. 2 MESI
I
aVR
V1
V4
II
aVL
V2
V5
III
aVF
V3
V6
150Hz
25.0mm/s
10.0mm/mV
4 x 2,5s
MAC5K 008B
12SL™v237

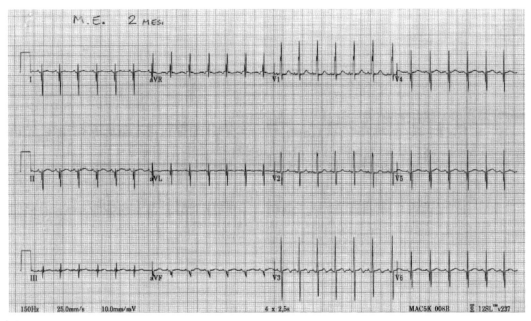

Fig. 3.3 Electrocardiogram recorded of a 2-month-old infant

In terms of the electrical activity of ventricular depolarization, the electrical forces of the ventricles are balanced in Fig. 3.3. In V_1, the R wave > S wave such that R/S > 1, and in V_6 the R wave > S wave such that R/S > 1. The voltage of the R wave in V_1 is 1.7 mV (17 mm) and the voltage of the S wave in V_6 is 0.8 mV (8 mm). These are both within normal limits. This trace therefore fits the "infant pattern", which is congruous with the age of this 2-month-old patient.

In V_1, there is also a slurring in the rise of the R wave in accordance with a slight intraventricular right conduction delay. The signs of right ventricular systolic overload are the positive T wave in V_1–V_2 and the approximately +200° right hyperdeviated QRS axis. The patient suffered from moderate congenital pulmonary valve stenosis.

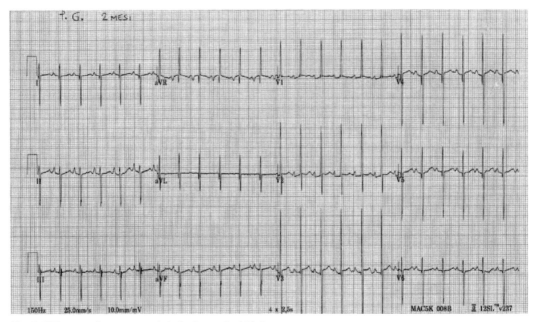

Fig. 3.4 Electrocardiogram recorded of a 2-month-old infant

This ECG is pathological due to the following signs of right ventricular hypertrophy (or right ventricular systolic overload). The clear electrical prevalence of the right ventricle fits the "neonatal pattern" and is incongruous with the age of this patient. This is visible in V_1 through the exclusive R wave with a voltage of 20 mm (2 mV), which far exceeds the maximum normal limit of 10 mm (1 mV). In V_6, the dominant S wave has a pathological voltage of 16 mm (1.6 mV) such that R/S < 1.

The positive T wave of ventricular repolarization in V_1–V_2 is pathological and indicates right ventricular systolic load. The strain and right QRS axis deviation (+220°) is also pathological. The patient suffered from a complete form of atrioventricular septal defect associated with pulmonary valve stenosis.

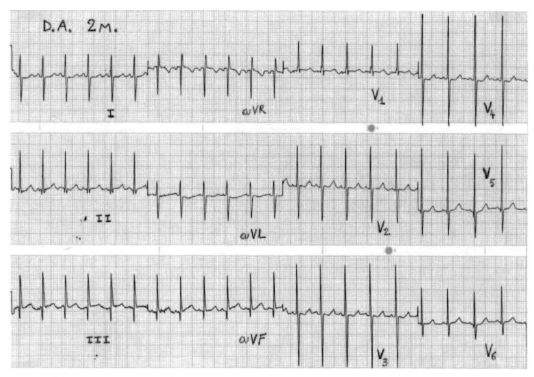

Fig. 3.5 Electrocardiogram recorded of a 2-month-old infant

With ventricular depolarization, the electrical forces of the ventricles are visibly balanced in this trace (Fig. 3.5). In V_1, the R wave > S wave so that R/S > 1 and in V_6 the R wave > S wave such that R/S > 1, making this fit the "infant pattern" which is congruous with the age of this 2-month-old patient.

The pathological element is the positive T wave of ventricular repolarization in V_1–V_2, which indicates right ventricular systolic overload. The +95° QRS frontal axis is normal. The patient suffered from Tetralogy of Fallot.

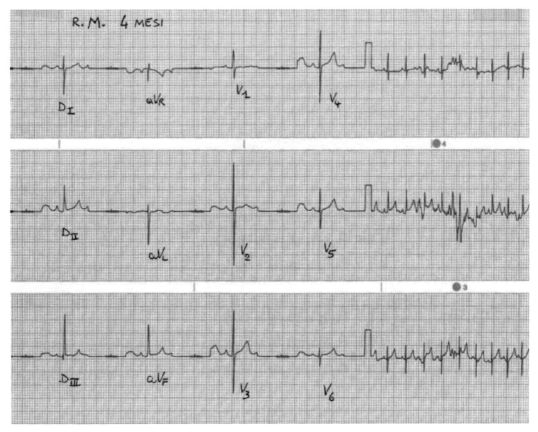

Fig. 3.6 Electrocardiogram recorded of a 4-month-old infant

In this trace (Fig. 3.6), the signs of right ventricular hypertrophy are evident in ventricular depolarization, which shows electrical prevalence of the right ventricle. Therefore, this ECG is consistent with the "neonatal pattern", which is inappropriate for the age of this 4-month-old patient. V_1 shows electrical dominance of the right ventricle where $R > S$ such that $R/S > 1$. In V_6, $S > R$ so $R/S < 1$.

The electrical activity of ventricular repolarization is also pathological since the T wave is positive in V_1–V_2, indicating right ventricular systolic overload. The QRS frontal axis however, is within normal limits since it is modestly right deviated at about +110°. The patient suffered from Tetralogy of Fallot.

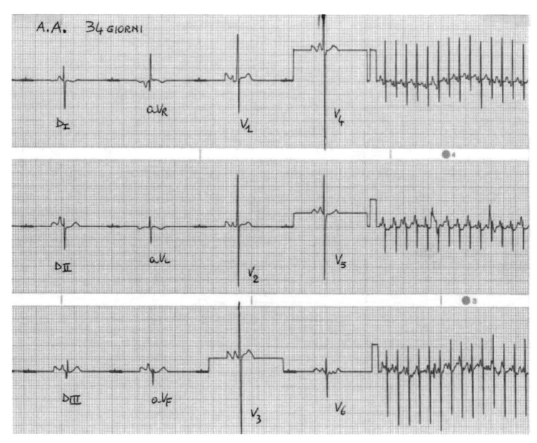

Fig. 3.7 Electrocardiogram recorded of a 34-day-old infant

As in Fig. 3.6, the sign of right ventricular hypertrophy here (Fig. 3.7) is electrical prevalence of the right ventricle, evident in ventricular depolarization. That means this is also consistent with the "neonatal pattern", which is inappropriate for the age of this patient, who is over a month old. As before, V_1 shows the electrical dominance of the right ventricle where R > S so R/S > 1, and in V_6, S > R such that R/S < 1.

Since the T wave is positive in V_1–V_2, the electrical activity of ventricular repolarization is also pathological, which indicates right ventricular systolic overload. The QRS frontal axis is pathologically right deviated at about +210°.

The patient suffered from a large muscular ventricular septal defect complicated by pulmonary arterial hypertension from a torrential pulmonary blood flow. Because of resistant heart failure, this defect required early surgical correction (in the second month of life).

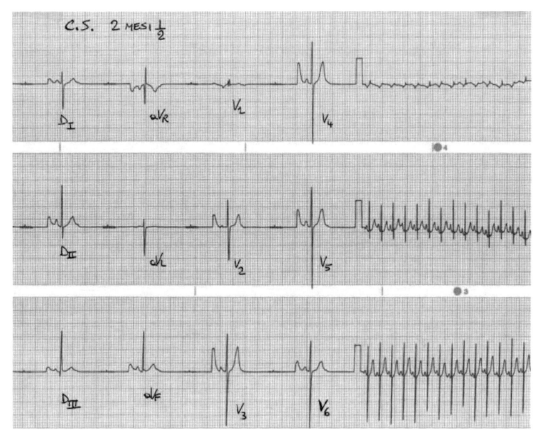

Fig. 3.8 Electrocardiogram recorded of a 2-month-old infant

Looking at the morphology of the QRS in the V_1 and V_6 precordial leads of Fig. 3.8, one can see the electrical prevalence of the right ventricle indicating the "neonatal pattern", which is inappropriate for the age of this patient. Therefore this ECG shows right ventricular hypertrophy. In V_6, a deep S wave (20 mm or 2 mV) of right ventricular depolarization is dominant over the R wave of left ventricular depolarization and has pathological voltage over the normal limit of 10 mm (1 mV) in that R/S < 1. The morphology of the QRS in V_1, however, is not pathological since the exclusive R wave has low voltage (2 mm or 0.2 mV), which is well within the normal limits.

The positive T wave of ventricular repolarization in V_1–V_2 is another sign of right ventricular systolic overload. The right axis deviation with the QRS frontal axis at +110° is within normal limits for the age of the patient.

The patient, in fact, suffered from a pulmonary outflow tract obstruction (Tetralogy of Fallot-type double-outlet right ventricle).

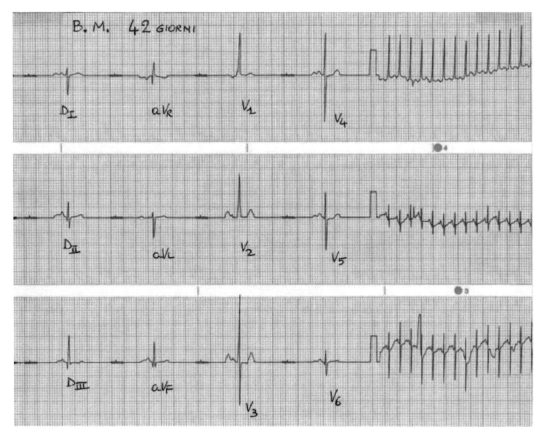

Fig. 3.9 Electrocardiogram recorded of a 42-day-old infant

The signs of right ventricular hypertrophy are evident in the precordial leads. In V_1, the pathological electrical prevalence of the right ventricle is shown by the exclusive R wave of right ventricular depolarization, which has a voltage of 16 mm (1.6 mV), which is higher than the 10 mm upper limit (see Table 1.1). In the V_6 precordial lead, the electrical dominance of the right ventricle, which is pathological given the age of the patient, has an R/S ratio of less than 1.

Another sign that confirms right ventricular systolic overload is the positive T wave in V_1–V_2.

The right axis deviation (+120°), which is within normal limits, does not add useful information for diagnosis. The patient suffered from infracardiac total anomalous pulmonary venous drainage associated with isthmic coarctation of the aorta with patent ductus arteriosus and severe pulmonary arterial hypertension.

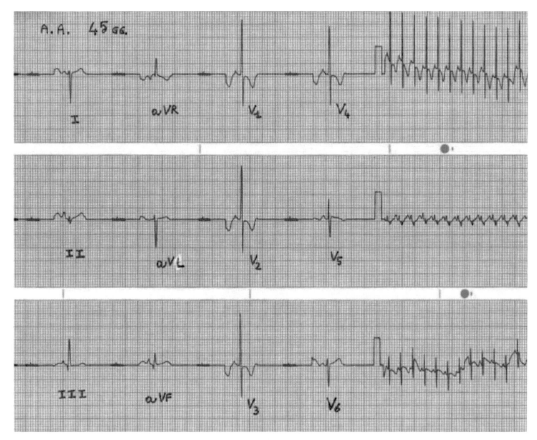

Fig. 3.10 Electrocardiogram recorded of a 45-day-old infant

With regard to ventricular depolarization, the sign of right ventricular hypertrophy in the V_1 and V_6 precordial leads is that the right ventricle is electrically dominant. This fits the "neonatal pattern" which is inappropriate for the age of this patient. In V_1, the right ventricle is prevalent so R > S such that R/S > 1. In V_6, S > R so R/S < 1.

For ventricular repolarization, the T wave is negative in V_1–V_2, which is normal and does not add to the pathological diagnosis. The QRS axis, however, is significantly right deviated at +160°, which indicates the pathological electrical dominance of the right ventricle. This patient suffered from infracardiac total anomalous pulmonary venous drainage.

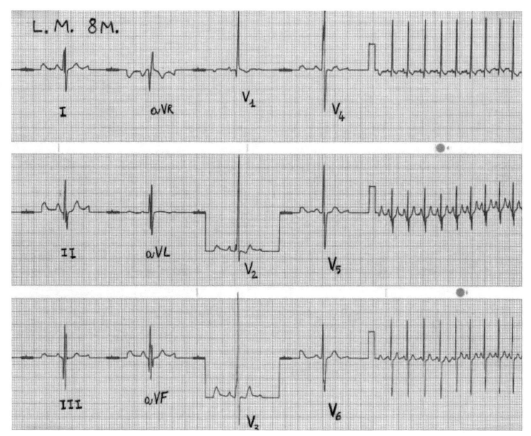

Fig. 3.11 Electrocardiogram recorded of an 8-month-old infant

The signs of right ventricular hypertrophy are visible in V_1 through a qR pattern where the pathological Q wave associated with the high voltage (2.2 mV) R wave indicates severe pressure and volume overload of the right ventricle. In V_6, it is visible through the R/S ratio that equals 1, with an S wave at a voltage of 1.3 mV (above the normal limit of 1 mV), which indicates the right ventricle's considerable electrical weight. This is altogether pathological for the age of the patient (8 months).

The pattern of ventricular repolarization is pathological due to the diphasic T wave in V_1–V_2–V_3. The +90° QRS axis, however, is within normal limits.

The patient suffered from a large ostium secundum-type atrial septal defect associated with patent ductus arteriosus complicated by severe pulmonary arterial hypertension.

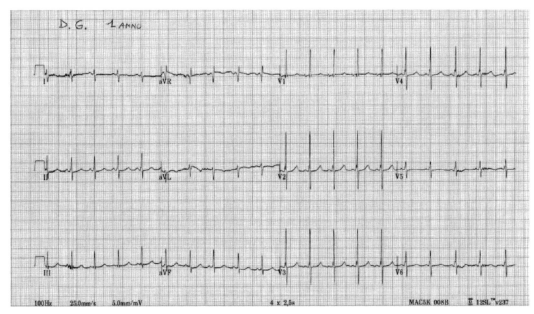

Fig. 3.12 Electrocardiogram recorded of a 1-year-old infant

In Fig. 3.12, the sign of right ventricular hypertrophy in V_1 is the exclusive R wave of ventricular depolarization with an amplitude of 14 mm (1.4 mV), which is above the normal limit of the "infant pattern" (see Table 1.3). In V_6, the pattern of ventricular depolarization is such that R/S > 1, so this does not add useful elements to the diagnosis of right ventricular hypertrophy. The pattern of ventricular repolarization indicates right ventricular systolic overload since the T wave is positive in V_1–V_2. The +100° QRS axis is within normal limits.

The patient suffered from left hypoplastic heart syndrome with systemic circulation supported by the dominant ventricle, which is morphologically right.

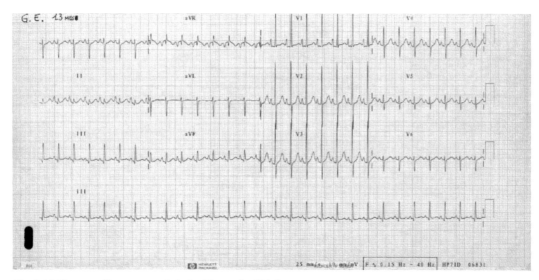

Fig. 3.13 Electrocardiogram recorded of a 13-month-old infant

Looking at the V_1 and V_6 precordial leads in Fig. 3.13, one can see the prevalence of the right ventricle in the electrical activity of ventricular depolarization. In V_1, the exclusive 20 mm (2 mV) R wave is pathological due to its voltage (see Table 1.1). In V_6, the right ventricle still prevails such that R/S < 1. This right ventricular prevalence defines the "neonatal pattern", which is incongruous with the age of this 13-month-old patient. Therefore, this ECG shows right ventricular hypertrophy corroborated by the pathological voltage of the R wave in V_1.

The electrical activity of ventricular repolarization indicates right ventricular systolic overload since the T wave is positive in V_1–V_2, which is pathological after the first week of life. The +130° QRS axis is sharply right deviated and is, therefore, pathological in relation to the age of the patient. It should be pointed out that, in V_1 and II leads, the 0.3 mV (3mm) voltage of the P wave of atrial depolarization indicates right atrial enlargement.

This ECG is, therefore, pathological due to signs of right ventricular systolic hypertrophy and overload. The patient suffered from Tetralogy of Fallot-type double-outlet right ventricle with Cornelia de Lange syndrome.

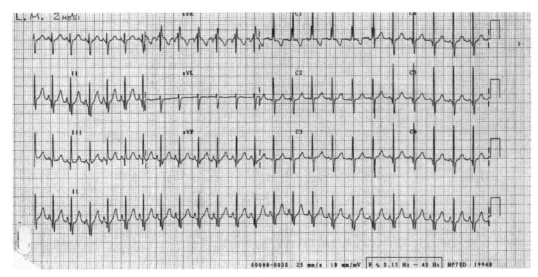

Fig. 3.14 Electrocardiogram recorded of a 2-month-old infant

The signs of right ventricular hypertrophy are visible in V_1 of Fig. 3.14, through an exclusive R wave of right ventricular depolarization with a voltage of 15 mm (1.5 mV), which is above the normal limit (see Table 1.3). Its morphology indicates right intraventricular electrical delay. In V_6, the pattern of ventricular depolarization is normal so R/S > 1.

Since the T wave is positive in V_2, the pattern of ventricular depolarization points to possible right ventricular systolic overload. The +110° right deviated QRS axis is normal for the age of this patient.

The patient suffered from a large perimembranous ventricular septal defect and pulmonary artery banding resulting from neonatal aortic decoarctation surgery.

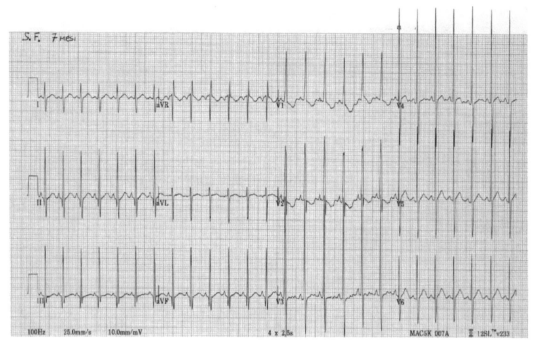

Fig. 3.15 Electrocardiogram recorded of a 7-month-old infant

In Fig. 3.15, the signs of right ventricular hypertrophy are visible in V_1 through an exclusive R wave of right ventricular depolarization with an amplitude of 25 mm (2.5 mV), which is above the normal limit (see Table 1.3). In V_6, the pattern of ventricular depolarization is congruous with the age of the patient with R/S > 1, but the amplitude of the S wave (12 mm or 1.2 mV) is above the normal limit of 1 mV. This confirms a pathological "electrical weight" of the right ventricle in relation to the age of the patient and a diagnosis of right ventricular hypertrophy.

Regarding ventricular repolarization, the morphology of the negative T wave in V_1–V_2 points to possible subendocardial ischemia within a context of right ventricular overload. The +90° QRS axis is within normal limits.

The patient suffered from severe bronchodysplasia due to prematurity associated with a mid-sized ostium secundum-type atrial septal defect.

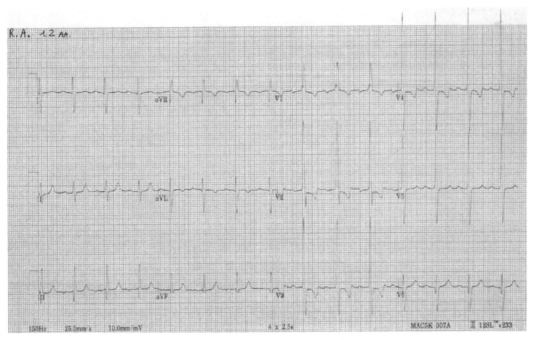

Fig. 3.16 Electrocardiogram recorded of a 12-year-old child

The signs of right ventricular hypertrophy are visible in the precordial leads of Fig. 3.16. In V_1, the pathological electrical prevalence of the right ventricle is evident through the exclusive R wave of ventricular depolarization that has a voltage of 14 mm (1.4 mV). This is always considered pathological after the age of 1. In the V_6 precordial lead, the right ventricle is electrically dominant such that R/S < 1 with the S wave's voltage at 1.2 mV. This "neonatal pattern" is pathological in relation to the age of the patient. Also, in V_1 the QRS morphology shows a slight right intraventricular electrical delay.

The T wave of ventricular repolarization is normal since it is negative in V_1–V_2 and positive in V_5–V_6. The QRS frontal axis is right deviated to +125°, which is pathological for the age of this patient and indicates right ventricular hypertrophy. The 230 ms PR interval indicates first degree atrioventricular block.

The patient suffered from hypoplastic left heart syndrome palliated with the Norwood operation.

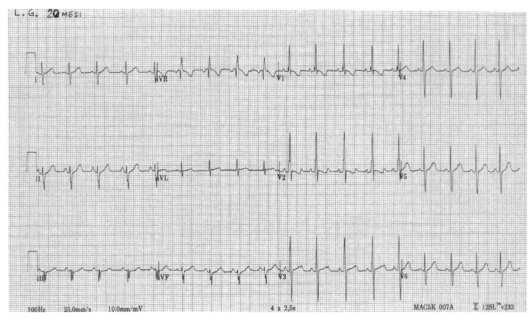

Fig. 3.17 Electrocardiogram recorded of a 20-month-old child

In Fig. 3.17, the morphology of the V_1 and V_6 precordial leads shows the right ventricle is electrically prevalent in ventricular depolarization. In V_1, the morphology of the QRS complex indicates a right intraventricular conduction delay and the R wave voltage is 13 mm (1.3 mV) wide. In V_6, the S wave magnitude is 8 mm (0.8 mV) such that R/S = 1. This is a sign that the electrical weight of the right ventricle is large enough to equal the weight of the left ventricle, which is pathological in V_6 for the age of this patient.

The right ventricle's electrical prevalence fits the "neonatal pattern", which is incongruous with the age of this 20-month-old patient and indicates right ventricular hypertrophy or enlargement, that is, systolic load associated with signs of right volume overload.

The electrical activity of ventricular repolarization is within normal limits since the T wave is negative in V_1, diphasic in V_2 and positive in V_5–V_6. This adds no useful information for diagnosis. The approximate -90° QRS frontal axis is, however, pathologically left hyperdeviated.

The patient suffered from a large hemodynamically significant ostium secundum-type atrial septal defect associated with moderate pulmonary valve stenosis.

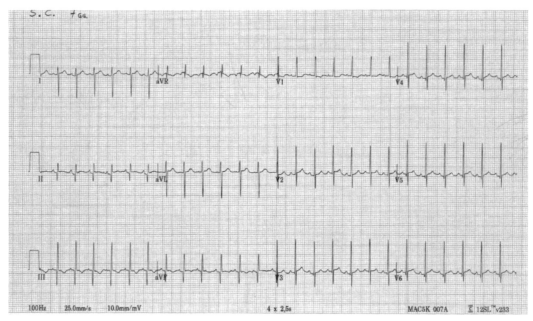

Fig. 3.18 Electrocardiogram recorded of a 7-day-old newborn

Looking at the V_1 and V_6 precordial leads in Fig. 3.18, one can see that the electrical forces of the ventricles are balanced. This fits the "infant pattern", which is a variation of the norm in the first month of life. In V_1, the 1 mV voltage of the exclusive R wave is within normal limits (see Table 1.3).

Since the T wave is positive in V_2 and diphasic in V_1, the ventricular repolarization here signals possible right ventricular systolic load. The +140° QRS frontal axis is within the normal limits for the age of this patient.

In this trace, the pattern of ventricular repolarization can be the sole basis to suspect right ventricular systolic load. The patient suffered from supracardiac total anomalous pulmonary venous drainage.

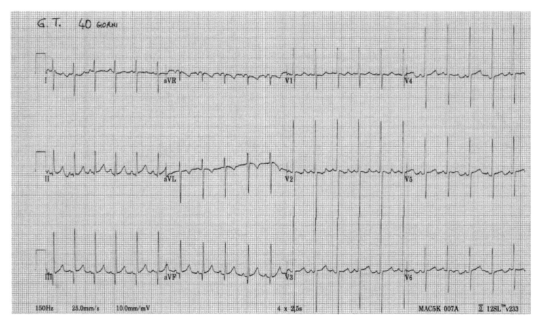

Fig. 3.19 Electrocardiogram recorded of a 40-day-old infant

In the V_1 and V_6 precordial leads of Fig. 3.19, one can see a pattern of balanced electrical forces in the ventricles such that R/S > 1 in each. In V_6, the S wave voltage at 10 mm is still at the upper limits of the norm, which is in accordance with the "infant pattern" and appropriate for the age of the patient. The +110° QRS frontal axis is also normal.

The element that indicates right ventricular systolic load is the morphology of ventricular repolarization since the T wave is positive in V_1 and diphasic in V_2. This patient suffered from Tetralogy of Fallot.

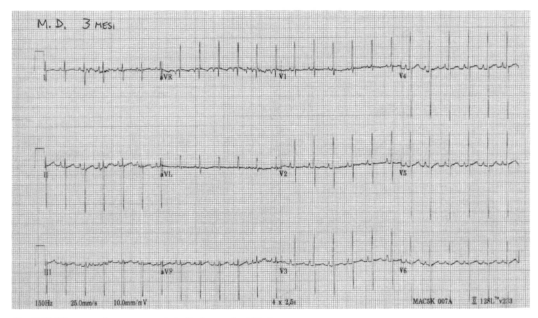

Fig. 3.20 Electrocardiogram recorded of a 3-month-old infant

When considering the electrical activity of ventricular depolarization in the V_1 and V_6 precordial leads (Fig. 3.20), the sign of right ventricular hypertrophy is the appearance of right ventricular prevalence, which fits the "neonatal pattern". This is pathological due to the fact that the patient is 3 months old. In V_1, the right ventricle is electrically dominant with R > S such that R/S > 1. In V_6, the electrical forces of the right ventricle are still prevalent with S > R so R/S < 1. The 20 mm voltage of the S wave surpasses by far the 10 mm upper limit of the norm and is thus pathological.

The morphology of ventricular repolarization indicates right ventricular systolic overload since the T wave is flat in V_1 and positive in V_2–V_3. The +230° QRS frontal axis is pathologically right hyperdeviated.

The patient suffered from a complete form of atrioventricular defect.

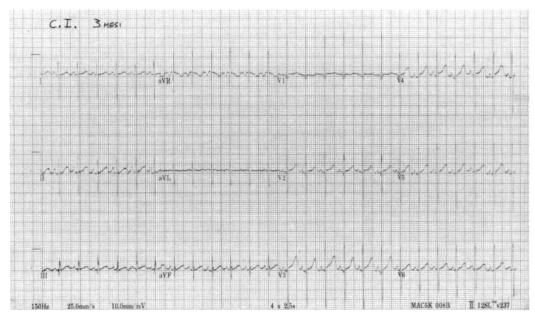

Fig. 3.21 Electrocardiogram recorded of a 3-month-old infant

In Fig. 3.21, signs of right ventricular hypertrophy are evident in the V_1 and V_6 precordial leads, which show right ventricular prevalence in ventricular depolarization. This is typical of the "neonatal pattern", but pathological in this case since the patient is 3 months old. In V_1, the 22 mm (2.2 mV) magnitude of the R wave is pathological since it surpasses the 20 mm normal limit. The miniscule Q wave is of note since it usually results from a severe pressure or volume overload of the right ventricle. In V_6, R/S < 1 and the pathological 14 mm S wave is greater than the 10 mm normal limit.

The morphology of ventricular repolarization indicates right ventricular systolic overload since the T wave is positive in V_1 and V_2. The +160° right deviated QRS frontal axis is pathological for the age of this patient.

The patient suffered from a large perimembranous ventricular septal defect associated with moderate pulmonary valve stenosis and with an ostium secundum-type atrial septal defect.

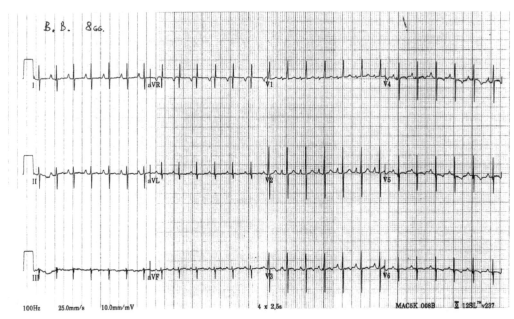

Fig. 3.22 Electrocardiogram recorded of an 8-day-old newborn

The "neonatal pattern" of right ventricular electrical prevalence is recognizable in Fig. 3.22, in V_1 through the 0.9 mV exclusive R wave, which is within normal limits (Table 1.1). It is also recognizable in V_6 through a well represented S wave such that R/S = 1. These elements are congruous with the age of this 8-day-old patient.

The morphology of ventricular repolarization points to possible right ventricular systolic load since the T wave is positive in V_1–V_2 and negative in V_3. The negative T wave in V_6 is normal considering the age of this patient.

The strain and left QRS frontal axis deviation (-70°) is pathological. In conclusion, even at only 8 days of life, this ECG suggests the signs of right ventricular load and should be considered pathological.

The patient suffered from an atrial septal defect associated with partial anomalous pulmonary venous drainage of the right pulmonary veins in the right atrium and severe pulmonary arterial hypertension.

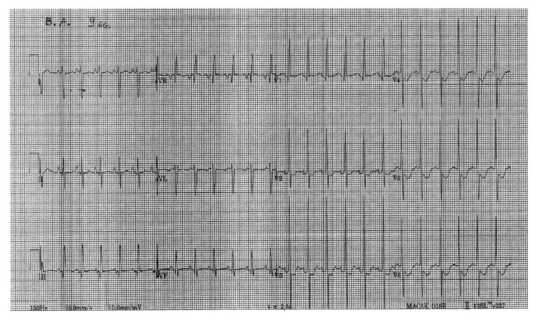

Fig. 3.23 Electrocardiogram recorded of a 9-day-old newborn

In V_1 of Fig. 3.23, signs of right ventricular hypertrophy are a qR pattern in which the Q wave indicates severe right ventricle pressure and volume overload, and an R wave with a 20 mm (2 mV) voltage, which is pathological since it is well above the 10 mm normal limit established after the first week of life. In V_6, the corroborating sign is the 1.5 mV voltage of the S wave, which is greater than the 1 mV limit. Otherwise, in V_6 the morphology of ventricular depolarization is in accord with the "infant pattern" (R/S > 1), which is a normal variant in the first month of life.

Here, the depression of the ST segment in the left precordial leads (3 mm from V_3 to V_6) is a stark sign of the pathology of the ventricular repolarization, which reflects myocardial ischemia. Moreover, the flat T wave in V_1 is compatible with right ventricular load. The +145° QRS frontal axis is within the normal limits for the first month of life. The patient suffered from a large coronary arterial fistula between the right coronary artery and the right atrium.

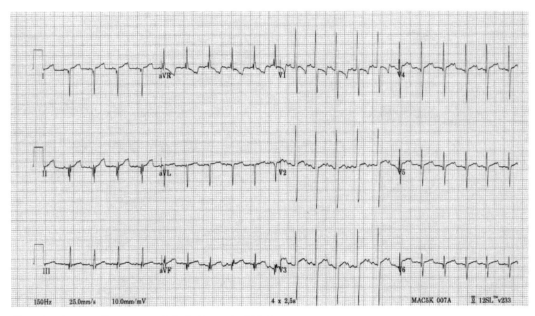

Fig. 3.24 Electrocardiogram recorded of a 7-month-old infant

In this trace (Fig. 3.24), the signs of right ventricular hypertrophy are visible in the electrical activity of ventricular depolarization. In V_1, the right ventricle is electrically dominant (R > S) such that R/S > 1. In V_6, the S wave prevails over the R wave, hence R/S < 1 with the appearance of right ventricular prevalence. This fits the "neonatal pattern" which is incongruous with the age of this 7-month-old patient. The markedly (+170°) right deviated QRS frontal axis is pathological.

Since the T wave is negative in V_1, ventricular repolarization shows normal morphology there, but since it is positive in V_2–V_3, this suggests possible right ventricular systolic load. The patient suffered from pulmonary valve stenosis.

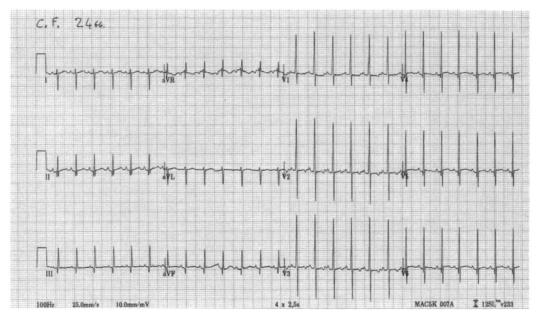

Fig. 3.25 Electrocardiogram recorded of a 24-day-old newborn

In Fig. 3.25, the morphology of ventricular depolarization in the V_1 and V_6 precordial leads shows that the electrical forces of the ventricles are balanced. This fits the "infant pattern" which is a variant of the norm in the first month of life and thus, appropriate for the age of this 24-day-old patient. In V_1, however, the 2 mV voltage of the R wave is at the upper limits of the norm. This is associated with the flat T wave of ventricular repolarization. These both suggest possible right ventricular systolic load. The +120° QRS frontal axis is normal.

In this ECG it is possible to detect signs that point to possible right ventricular systolic load. The patient suffered from moderate pulmonary valve stenosis.

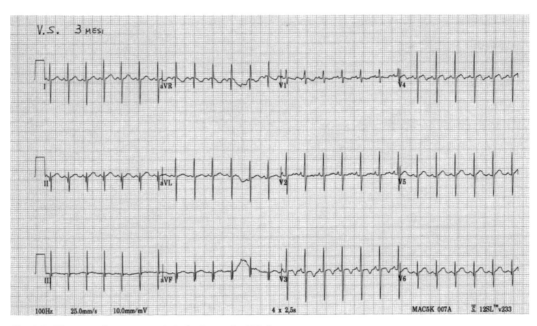

V.S.   3 MESI

100Hz   25.0mm/s   10.0mm/mV   4 x 2,5s   MAC5K 007A   Σ 12SL™v233

Fig. 3.26 Electrocardiogram recorded of a 3-month-old infant

In Fig. 3.26, the "neonatal pattern" of right ventricular prevalence is visible in V_6 since the S wave > the R wave such that R/S < 1. This is incongruous with the age of this 3-month-old infant and thus indicates right ventricular hypertrophy.

The +170° right deviated QRS frontal axis is also pathological. The morphology of ventricular repolarization is essentially normal since the T wave is negative in V_1 and positive in V_6. The patient suffered from a large ostium secundum-type atrial septal defect associated with patent ductus arteriosus.

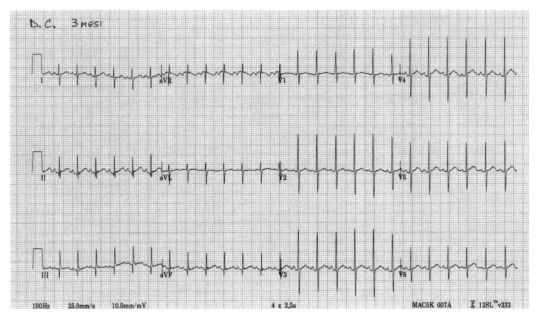

Fig. 3.27 Electrocardiogram recorded of a 3-month-old infant

Looking at the morphology of ventricular depolarization in the V_1 and V_6 precordial leads, one can see that the electrical forces of the ventricles are balanced (in V_1, R wave > S wave such that R/S > 1; in V_6, R wave > S wave in that R/S > 1). This is normal since it fits the "infant pattern" and is appropriate for the age of this 3-month-old patient. The +95° QRS frontal axis is also normal. The sign of a pathological condition in this ECG is the T wave of ventricular repolarization, which is positive in V_1–V_2, and points to possible right ventricular systolic load.

In this ECG, it is possible to detect signs indicating right ventricular systolic load based solely on the morphology of ventricular repolarization. The patient suffered from a large ostium secundum-type atrial septal defect associated with Down's syndrome.

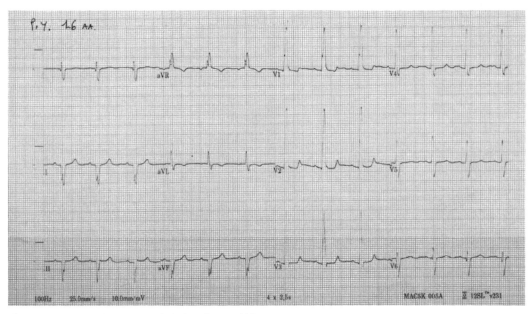

Fig. 3.28 Electrocardiogram recorded of a 16-year-old boy

The signs of right ventricular hypertrophy are evident in the precordial leads of Fig. 3.28. In V_1, the pattern of right ventricular depolarization is the qR type where the Q wave indicates severe pressure and volume overload of the right ventricle. This is associated with the exclusive R wave with a voltage of 22 mm (2.2 mV), which is always considered pathological after the age of 1. In the V_6 precordial lead, the electrical prevalence of the right ventricle shows a ratio of R/S < 1. This is pathological in relation to the age of the patient. The 0.9 mV voltage of the S wave is over the normal limit of 0.5 mV after the age of 3. Moreover, the QRS duration is 120 ms, which indicates a complete right bundle branch block type, right intraventricular electrical delay.

The QRS frontal axis is +250° right hyperdeviated, and thus is pathological. The morphology of ventricular repolarization is normal since the T wave is diphasic in V_1–V_2 and positive in V_5–V_6. This adds no useful elements for diagnosis.

The patient suffered from a morphologically right univentricular heart with mitral atresia and double outlet, palliated with a bidirectional cavopulmonary anastomosis (modified Glenn) and Fontan repair.

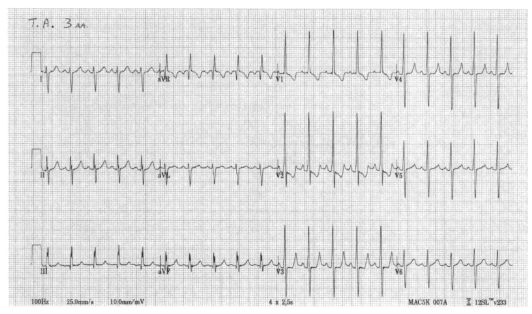

T. A. 3 m.

Fig. 3.29 Electrocardiogram recorded of a 3-year-old child

Looking at the precordial leads in Fig. 3.29, in V_1 one can see a high voltage (2.2 mV) exclusive R wave of right ventricular depolarization, which is entirely pathological for a 3 year old. In V_6, the electrical forces of the right ventricle are dominant such that R/S < 1. These elements fit the "neonatal pattern", which is pathological in terms of the age of this patient, and therefore indicates a diagnosis of right ventricular hypertrophy.

In V_1 and V_2, inverted T-waves suggest subendocardial ischemia within a context of right systolic overload. The +150° QRS frontal axis is pathologically right deviated with regards to the age of the patient. The patient suffered from partial anomalous pulmonary venous drainage associated with atrial septal superior sinus venosus defect and severe pulmonary arterial hypertension.

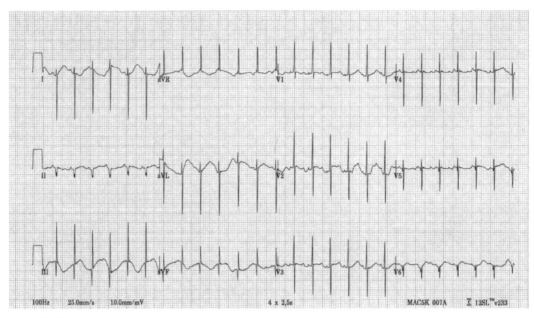

Fig. 3.30 Electrocardiogram recorded of a 2-month-old infant

In the V_1 and V_6 precordial leads of Fig. 3.30, one can see that the right ventricle's electrical forces of depolarization are dominant such that in V_6, the R wave of left ventricular depolarization is absent. This fits the "neonatal pattern", which is incongruous with the age of the patient and thus endorses the diagnosis of right ventricular hypertrophy.

The morphology of ventricular repolarization also indicates right ventricular systolic load since the T wave is positive in V_1, V_2 and V_3. At a marked +170° right deviation, the QRS frontal axis is also pathological after the first month of life. The patient suffered from severe pulmonary valve stenosis.

3.2 Right Ventricular Diastolic Overload

Right ventricular diastolic overload refers to an overload of volume in the right ventricle, i.e. the right ventricle pumps a stroke volume larger than the left ventricle.

This hemodynamic condition is found in congenital cardiopathies characterized by pretricuspid left to right shunts, for example, atrial septal defects, or total or partial anomalous pulmonary venous drainage. It is recognized at the echocardiography by enlargement of the right ventricle associated with paradox movement of the ventricular septum. On the ECG, there will be a pattern of delay in conduction along the right bundle branch in V_1, which typically has an rSR' pattern such that R' > r and the T wave is negative. These elements can be accompanied by a right deviated QRS frontal axis (see Table 3.2).

The rSR' pattern in which R' > r always suggests right ventricular enlargement secondary to a congenital cardiopathy and is distinct from the RSr'-type incomplete right bundle branch block. The latter, common among normal newborns and infants, generally represents a simple right intraventricular conduction delay.

Table 3.2 Right ventricular diastolic overload or volume overload

In V_1	rSR' pattern such that R' > r
	Negative T wave
QRS frontal axis > +120°	

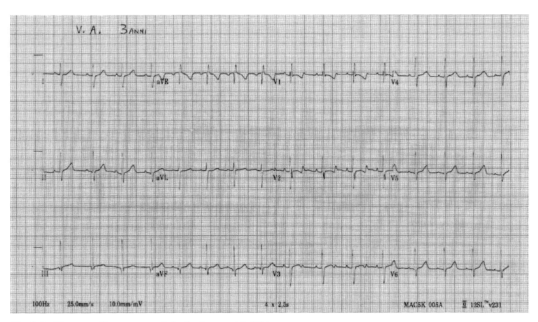

Fig. 3.31 Electrocardiogram recorded of a 3-year-old child

In the V_1 precordial lead of Fig. 3.31, one can see a pattern of incomplete right bundle branch block such that R' > r, which indicates right ventricle volume overload. In the V_6 precordial lead, the electrical forces of the left ventricle are prevalent which is normal for a patient of this age.

Since the T wave is negative in V_1–V_2, the morphology of ventricular repolarization is also normal. The +90° QRS frontal axis is normal as well.

In conclusion, the only pathological sign in this trace is incomplete right bundle branch block such that R' > r, indicating right ventricle volume overload. The patient, in fact, suffered from a hemodynamically significant ostium secundum-type atrial septal defect.

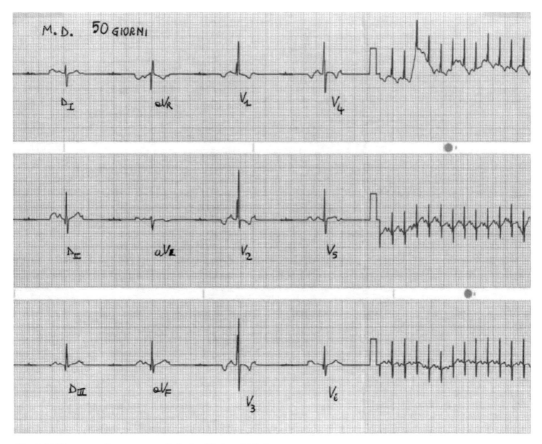

Fig. 3.32 Electrocardiogram recorded of a 50-day-old infant

In Fig. 3.32, the pathological aspect in the V_1 precordial lead is the high voltage (12 mm, 1.2 mV) exclusive R wave, which is above the 1 mV normal limit. This indicates right ventricular hypertrophy due to pressure overload. The presence of a notch on the ascending branch of the R wave is indicative of a possible volume overload. In the V_6 precordial lead, the R wave of left ventricular depolarization is electrically dominant which fits the "infant pattern" and is normal.

The morphology of ventricular repolarization fits the "infant pattern" as well since the T wave is negative in V_1, V_2, V_3 and V_4. The QRS frontal axis is slightly right deviated at $+110°$, which is within normal limits for the age of this patient.

The patient suffered from an ostium secundum-type atrial septal defect associated with left cor triatriatum complicated by pulmonary arterial hypertension.

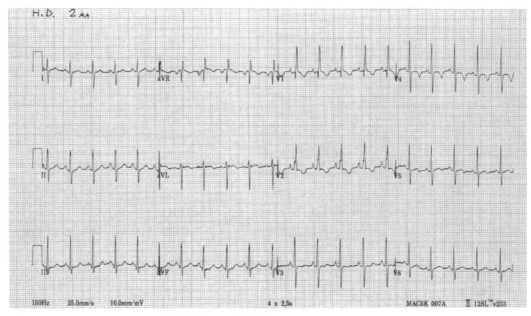

Fig. 3.33 Electrocardiogram recorded of a 2-year-old child

In the V_1 precordial lead, one can see an rSR' aspect where the pattern of incomplete right bundle branch block (in which R' > r) indicates right ventricular volume overload (Fig. 3.33). In the V_6 precordial lead, the electrical forces of the left ventricle are prevalent in that R/S > 1, which is normal for a patient of this age.

The morphology of ventricular repolarization is normal since the T wave is negative in V_1–V_2. The QRS frontal axis is slightly right deviated at +120°, which is above the +100° normal limit for this age.

In conclusion, the elements in this ECG that point to a possible pathological condition are the slight right deviation of the QRS axis and the pattern of incomplete right bundle branch block such that R' > r, which indicates right ventricular volume overload. In fact the patient suffered from a large hemodynamically significant ostium secundum-type atrial septal defect.

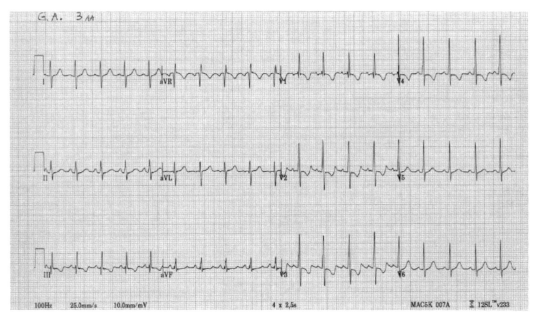

Fig. 3.34 Electrocardiogram recorded of a 3-year-old child

In Fig. 3.34, the V_1 precordial lead has an rSR' aspect where the pattern of incomplete right bundle branch block (R' > r) suggests right ventricular volume overload. In the V_6 precordial lead, the electrical forces of the left ventricle are prevalent such that R/S > 1, which is normal for a patient of this age. The morphology of ventricular repolarization is normal since the T wave is negative in V_1–V_2–V_3. The +85° QRS frontal axis is also normal.

In summary, the only element in this ECG that indicates a pathogical condition is the aspect of incomplete right bundle branch block such that R' > r, which indicates right ventricular volume overload. The patient suffered from a hemodynamically significant superior sinus venosus atrial septal defect.

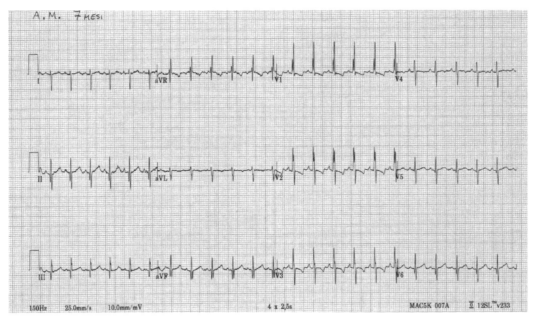

Fig. 3.35 Electrocardiogram recorded of a 7-month-old infant

In the V_1 precordial lead of Fig. 3.35, one can see the infant pattern with an R/S > 1 ratio, which shows a high R wave with a notch on the ascending branch. This indicates a delay in right intraventricular conduction suggesting right ventricle volume overload. In the V_6 precordial lead, the electrical forces of the left ventricle are prevalent such that R/S > 1, which fits the "infant pattern" and is normal for a patient of this age.

The morphology of ventricular repolarization is normal since the T wave is negative in V_1–V_2–V_3. The QRS frontal axis is pathologically right deviated at +150°, which is above the +120° normal limit for this age.

In this ECG, the right deviation of the QRS axis and the pattern of incomplete right bundle branch block indicate a pathological condition. The patient suffered from a large hemodynamically significant ostium secundum-type atrial septal defect.

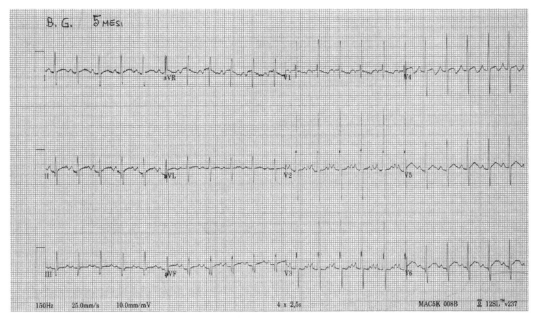

Fig. 3.36 Electrocardiogram recorded of a 5-month-old infant

In Fig. 3.36, the V_1 precordial lead has a pattern of incomplete right bundle branch block (in which R' > r), indicating right ventricular volume overload. In the V_6 precordial lead, the electrical forces of the left ventricle are prevalent such that R/S > 1 and the 0.7 mV S wave of right ventricular depolarization is within the 1 mV normal limit. These elements fit the "infant pattern" and are appropriate for the age of the patient.

Considering the morphology of ventricular repolarization, the T wave is negative in V_1, which is normal, but positive in V_2–V_3, which points to possible right ventricle systolic load. The +65° QRS frontal axis is normal.

In this trace the elements pointing to a pathological condition are the positive T wave in V_2–V_3 and the pattern of incomplete right bundle branch block (in which R' > r), indicating right ventricular volume overload. The patient suffered from a large hemodynamically significant ostium secundum-type atrial septal defect.

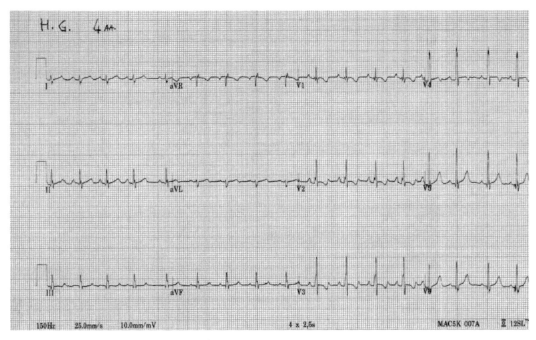

Fig. 3.37 Electrocardiogram recorded of a 4-year-old child

In the V_1 precordial lead of Fig. 3.37, one can see a pattern of incomplete right bundle branch block (in which R' > r) indicating right ventricular volume overload. In the V_6 precordial lead, the electrical forces of the left ventricle are prevalent such that R/S > 1, normal for the patient's age.

The morphology of ventricular repolarization is normal since the T wave is negative in V_1–V_2–V_3. The +70° QRS frontal axis is also normal.

In this ECG, the only element pointing to a pathologic condition is the pattern of incomplete right bundle branch block (in which R' > r), indicating right ventricular volume overload. The patient suffered from a large ostium secundum-type atrial septal defect.

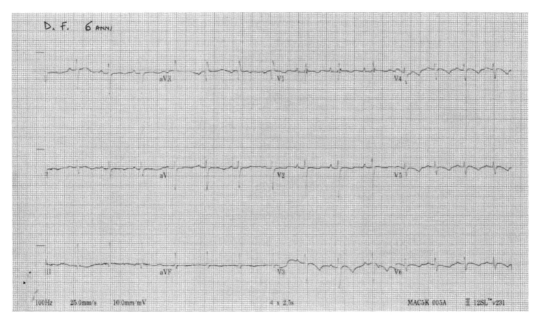

Fig. 3.38 Electrocardiogram recorded of a 6-year-old child

Considering the precordial leads, the pattern of ventricular depolarization in V_1 (Fig. 3.38) points to right ventricular volume overload due to the R' > r type incomplete right bundle branch block. In V_6, the voltage of the S wave of right ventricular depolarization is equal to that of the R wave of left ventricular depolarization such that R/S = 1. Since there is no electrical prevalence of the left ventricle, this ECG shows pathological right ventricle dominance.

The pattern of ventricular repolarization is pathological since the T wave is diphasic in V_1–V_2 and negative from V_3 to V_6. Analogously, the QRS frontal axis is right deviated at +150°, which is above the normal limit of +100° for the age of this patient.

These elements make up a pathological trace that shows right ventricular volume and pressure overload. The patient suffered from a large hemodynamically significant ostium secundum-type atrial septal defect with moderate pulmonary arterial hypertension.

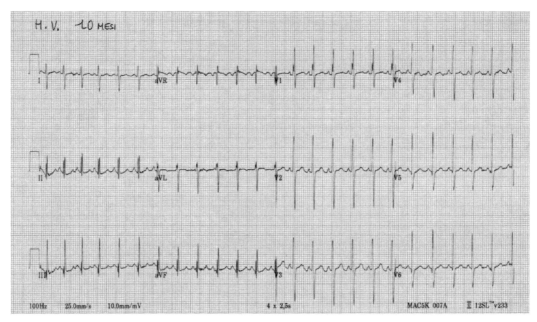

Fig. 3.39 Electrocardiogram recorded of a 10-month-old infant

In the V_1 precordial lead, the "infant pattern", with an R/S > 1 ratio, shows an R wave with a notch on the ascending branch, which indicates a right intraventricular conduction delay suggesting right ventricular volume overload. In the V_6 precordial lead, the electrical forces of the left ventricle are prevalent. The S wave of right ventricular depolarization has a voltage of 0.9 mV, which is within the 1 mV normal limit. The ratio of the R wave to the S wave is R/S > 1. These elements fit the "infant pattern", which is normal for the age of this patient.

The morphology of ventricular repolarization indicates right ventricular systolic load since the T wave is positive in V_1–V_2–V_3. The +115° QRS frontal axis is normal for the age of the patient.

In this ECG, the pattern of an incomplete right bundle branch block and the positive T wave in V_1–V_2–V_3 indicate a pathological condition. The patient suffered from a large hemodynamically significant ostium secundum-type atrial septal defect with moderate pulmonary arterial hypertension.

Left Ventricular Overload

4

4.1 Left Ventricular Systolic and Diastolic Overload

In the left ventricle, left ventricular systolic and diastolic overload refer to pressure overload and volume overload. These two hemodynamic situations cause left ventricular hypertrophy and left ventricular dilatation respectively. From an electrocardiographical standpoint they can be considered together since they are both expressed by the same observation: the appearance of the "adult pattern" of left ventricular prevalence on an ECG, before the age of 2 and with the S and R wave's pathological voltage in V_1 and V_6 precordial leads.

Considering the V_1 and V_6 precordial leads, the ECG pattern shows the prevalence of the electrical forces of the left ventricle. In V_1, the S wave of left ventricular depolarization is dominant over the R wave of right ventricular depolarization such that R/S < 0.4 and the S wave > 20 mm (> 2 mV). In V_4, V_5 and V_6, the R wave of left ventricular depolarization not only dominates, but has high voltage such that R > 25 mm (> 2.5 mV).

Regarding the electrical activity of ventricular repolarization, it is necessary to look at the morphology of the T wave in the V_5 and V_6 precordial leads. The T wave will be positive if the volume overload prevails, and negative if the pressure overload prevails. These elements can be accompanied by a left deviated QRS frontal axis (see Table 4.1).

It is crucial to refer to the age of the patient when judging an abnormal electrocardiogram and making a diagnosis of left ventricular hypertrophy with signs of volume or pressure overload. In general the "adult pattern" is found after the age of 2; in younger patients, one must judge the "adult pattern" to be incongruous with the age of the patient, except in the cases that show the S and R wave's voltage within the normal limits. Before the age of 2, left ventricular prevalence points to possible left ventricular hypertrophy.

Table 4.1 Left ventricular pressure and volume overload. Left ventricular hypertrophy or enlargement is defined by the appearance of the "adult pattern" before the age of 2

In V_1	S wave > 20 mm
	R/S < 0.4
In V_4–V_5–V_6	high voltage R wave (R > 25 mm, 2.5 mV)
In V_5–V_6	positive/negative T wave
Left axial deviation	

M. A. Galli (✉)
Perinatal and Pediatric Cardiology
Ospedale Maggiore Policlinico
Milan, Italy
e-mail: mariellagalli@gmail.com

M. A. Galli, G. B. Danzi, *A Guide to Neonatal and Pediatric ECGs*,
DOI: 10.1007/978-88-470-2856-2_4, © Springer-Verlag Italia 2013

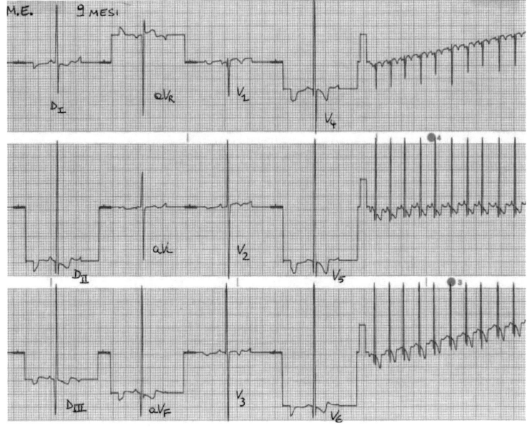

Fig. 4.1 Electrocardiogram rcorded of a 9-month-old infant

Considering the V_1 and V_6 precordial leads (Fig. 4.1), one can see that the left ventricle is prevalent in the electrical activity of ventricular depolarization. This fits the "adult pattern", which is incongruous with the age of the patient. In V_1, the S wave of left ventricular depolarization is dominant in that R/S < 0.4. In V_4, V_5 and V_6, the R wave of left ventricular depolarization is dominant and has a high voltage of 45 mm or 4.5 mV, which exceeds the normal limit of 2.5 mV.

In terms of ventricular repolarization, the negative T wave in V_5–V_6 is pathological. These elements constitute a picture of severe left ventricular enlargement. The +70° QRS frontal axis is normal. This patient presented with a severe dilated cardiomyopathy of the left ventricle.

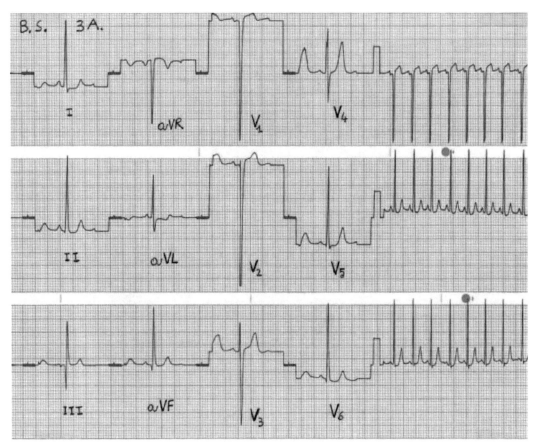

Fig. 4.2 Electrocardiogram recorded of a 3-year-old child

In this case (Fig. 4.2), the "adult pattern", although appropriate for the age of the patient, is pathological due to signs of left ventricular hypertrophy. In V_1, the very deep S wave of left ventricular depolarization (45 mm, 4.5 mV) is far higher than the normal limit of 2 mV. In V_6, the R wave of left ventricular depolarization has pathological voltage at 28 mm or 2.8 mV. The pattern of ventricular repolarization is pathological since the T wave is diphasic in the V_6 lateral chest lead and in the I–aV_L extremity leads.

These elements constitute a picture of left ventricular hypertrophy-overload. The +50° QRS frontal axis is normal. The patient suffered from an obstructive hypertrophic cardiomyopathy of the left ventricle.

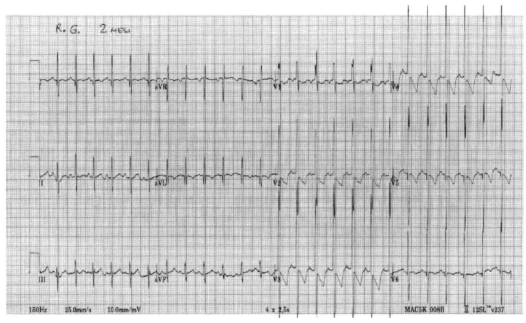

Fig. 4.3 Electrocardiogram recorded of a 2-month-old infant

Looking at the V_1 and V_6 precordial leads in Fig. 4.3, we find that the electrical forces are balanced, which fits the "infant pattern" and is appropriate for the patient's age. In V_1, the R wave of right ventricular depolarization is dominant, so R/S > 1. In V_6, the R wave of left ventricular depolarization is dominant such that R/S > 1. The pathological elements in this trace are the +10° left deviated QRS axis and the high voltage of the R wave in V_4 (4 mV), V_5 (3.5 mV) and V_6 (2.5 mV), which are compatible with left ventricular hypertrophy.

The pattern of ventricular repolarization is normal in V_1–V_2–V_3 since the T wave is negative there, but in the V_5–V_6 lateral chest leads and in the I–aV_L high extremity leads, it is a sign of left ventricular overload since the T wave is also negative there.

These considerations constitute a pathological ECG picture that indicates left ventricular enlargement and overload. The patient suffered from a large hemodynamically significant perimembranous ventricular septal defect, which required surgical correction at the age of 3 months.

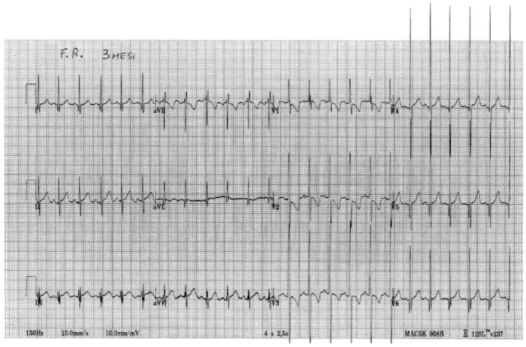

Fig. 4.4 Electrocardiogram recorded of a 3-month-old infant

The considerations made with the chart in Fig. 4.3 are also valid here (Fig. 4.4). In V_1 and V_6, we find the "infant pattern", which is appropriate for the patient's age. The pathological elements in this trace are the $+10°$ left deviated QRS axis and the high voltage of the R wave in V_4 (5.5 mV), V_5 (4.5 mV) and V_6 (2.7 mV), which is compatible with left ventricular hypertrophy.

The pattern of ventricular repolarization is normal in V_1–V_2–V_3 since the T wave is negative there, and normal in the V_5–V_6 lateral chest leads and in the I extremity lead, since the T wave is positive there.

These considerations constitute a pathological ECG picture that is compatible with left ventricular enlargement due to volume overload. The patient suffered from a large hemodynamically significant muscular ventricular septal defect, which required cardiac therapy.

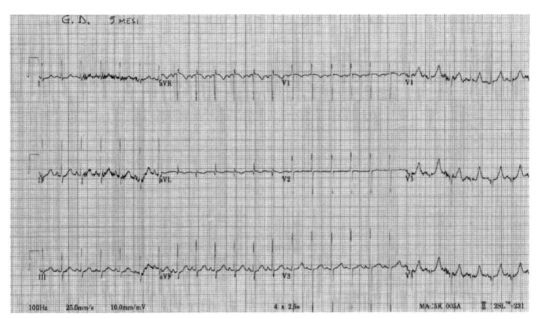

Fig. 4.5 Electrocardiogram recorded of a 5-month-old infant

In the electrical activity of ventricular depolarization in the V_1 and V_6 precordial leads (Fig. 4.5), one can see the electrical prevalence of the left ventricle. This fits the "adult pattern", which is incongruous with the age of the patient. In V_1, the S wave of left ventricular depolarization is dominant such that R/S < 0.4. In V_4, V_5 and V_6, the R wave of left ventricular depolarization is dominant and has a pathologically high voltage (> 2.5 mV).

In terms of the electrical activity of ventricular repolarization, the pathological aspect is less clear since the T wave slightly hints at negativity initially in V_6, while it is normal (negative) in V_1.

These elements constitute the pathological picture of left ventricular hypertrophy and initial overload. The +60° QRS frontal axis is still, however, within the limits of the norm. The patient suffered from severe supravalvular aortic stenosis in a picture of Williams syndrome.

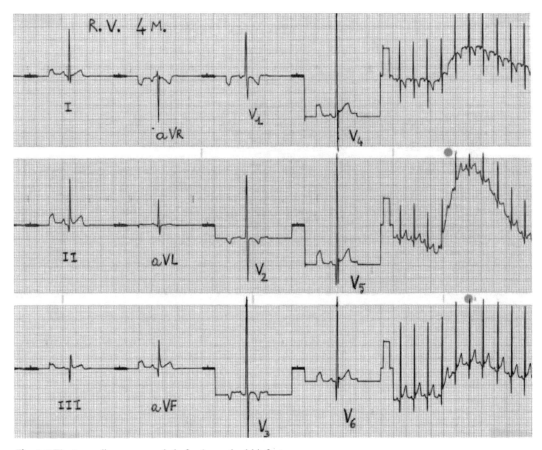

Fig. 4.6 Electrocardiogram recorded of a 4-month-old infant

Looking at the morphology of the V_1 and V_6 precordial leads in Fig. 4.6, we find the electrical forces of the ventricles are balanced. This fits the "infant pattern" which is appropriate for the age of the patient. In V_1, the R wave of right ventricular depolarization is dominant in that R/S > 1. In V_6, the R wave of left ventricular depolarization is dominant such that R/S > 1. The pathological elements in this ECG are the +20° left deviated QRS frontal axis and the high voltage of the R wave in V_4 (4 mV), V_5 (4.5 mV) and V_6 (3.5 mV), which is compatible with left ventricular hypertrophy.

The pattern of ventricular repolarization is normal in V_1–V_2–V_3 since the T wave is negative there, and normal in the V_5–V_6 lateral chest leads and in the I–aV_L extremity leads, since the T wave is positive there.

One can draw the conclusion that this ECG is pathological and indicates left ventricular enlargement due to volume overload. The patient suffered from a large hemodynamically significant perimembranous ventricular septal defect.

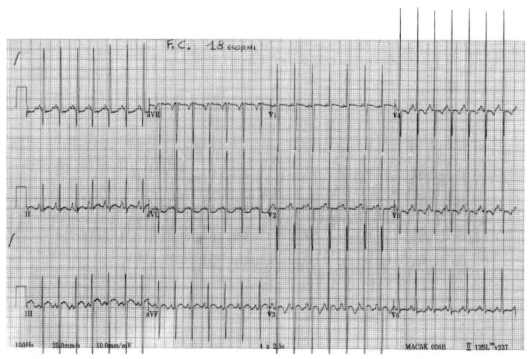

Fig. 4.7 Electrocardiogram recorded of an 18-day-old newborn

In the electrical activity of ventricular depolarization in the V_1 and V_6 precordial leads of Fig. 4.7, one can see the electrical prevalence of the left ventricle, which is incongruous with the age of the patient. In V_1, the deep (2.2 mV) S wave of left ventricular depolarization is equal in voltage to the R wave of right ventricular depolarization such that R/S = 1. This is pathological in the first month of life since both the "infant pattern" and the "neonatal pattern" include right ventricular electrical dominance. In V_6, the R wave of left ventricular depolarization has a high voltage of 2.1 mV, which rises to 5 mV in V_4 and V_5.

The pathological aspect in ventricular repolarization is the T wave, which is flat in V_1–V_2, and negative in V_5–V_6 and the I–aV_L leads. The QRS frontal axis is also left deviated at -10°. These elements constitute a pathological picture of left ventricular hypertrophy-overload.

The patient suffered from morphologically left univentricular heart with absent right atrioventricular connection.

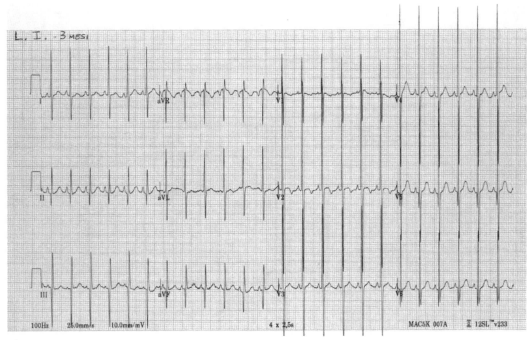

Fig. 4.8 Electrocardiogram recorded of a 3-month-old infant

Looking at the morphology of the V_1 and V_6 precordial leads in Fig. 4.8, we find that the electrical forces are balanced, which fits the "infant pattern" and is appropriate for the patient's age. In V_1, the R wave of right ventricular depolarization is dominant in that R/S > 1. In V_6, the R wave of left ventricular depolarization is dominant such that R/S > 1. The pathological elements in this trace are the high voltage of the R wave in V_4 (4.5 mV), V_5 (5 mV) and V_6 (3 mV) precordial leads and the +15° left deviated QRS frontal axis, which are all compatible with a diagnosis of left ventricular hypertrophy.

In the III lead, the deep and narrow Q wave presents a pathological voltage that exceeds the normal limit of 10 mm or 1 mV. The pattern of ventricular repolarization is normal in V_1–V_2 since the T wave is negative there. It is also normal in the V_5–V_6 lateral chest leads and in the I–aV_L extremity leads since the T wave is positive there. In this context, however, this is a sign of left ventricular volume overload.

These observations constitute a pathological ECG picture that indicates left ventricular hypertrophy and diastolic overload. The patient suffered from a large, restrictive, hemodynamically significant perimembranous ventricular septal defect.

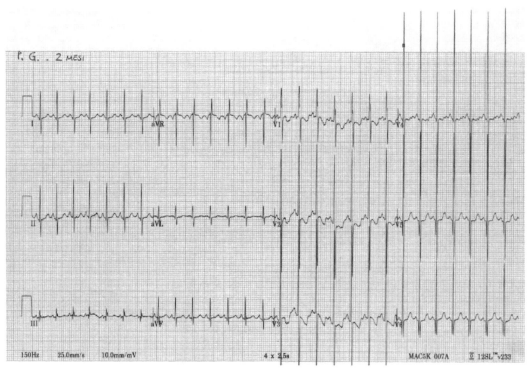

Fig. 4.9 Electrocardiogram recorded of a 2-month-old infant

Looking at the V_1 and V_6 precordial leads in Fig. 4.9, we find that the electrical forces of the ventricles are balanced, which fits the "infant pattern" and is appropriate for the patient's age. In V_1, the R wave of right ventricular depolarization is dominant such that R/S > 1. In V_6, the R wave of left ventricular depolarization is dominant such that R/S > 1. The pathological elements in this trace are the +45° left tending QRS axis and the high voltage of the R wave in V_4 (5 mV), V_5 (4.5 mV) and V_6 (3 mV), which are compatible with left ventricular hypertrophy.

The pattern of ventricular repolarization is normal in V_1–V_2–V_3 since the T wave is negative there. It is also normal in the V_5–V_6 lateral chest leads and in the I–aV_L extremity leads since the T wave is positive there. In this context, however, this is a sign of left ventricular volume overload.

It can be concluded that this ECG presents a pathological picture of left ventricular enlargement due to volume overload. The patient suffered from a large, restrictive, hemodynamically significant perimembranous ventricular septal defect.

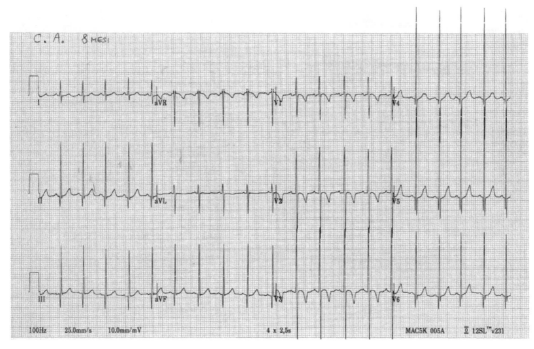

Fig. 4.10 Electrocardiogram recorded of an 8-month-old infant

For Fig. 4.10, when considering the morphology of the V_1 and V_6 precordial leads, one can see that the left ventricle is prevalent in the electrical activity of ventricular depolarization. This suggests left ventricular enlargement. In V_1, the S wave of left ventricular depolarization is dominant such that R/S < 1. In V_6, the R wave of left ventricular depolarization is dominant and has a high voltage of 3 mV, which grows to 4.5 mV in V_4 and V_5. These values exceed the normal limit of 2.5 mV.

The pattern of ventricular repolarization is normal in V_1–V_2–V_3 since the T wave is negative there. It is also normal in the V_5–V_6 lateral chest leads and in the I–aV_L extremity lead since the T wave is positive there. In this context, however, this is a sign of left ventricular volume overload. The +75° QRS frontal axis is normal.

It can be concluded that this is a pathological ECG picture that indicates left ventricular enlargement due to volume overload. The patient suffered from a large, restrictive, hemodynamically significant patent ductus arteriosus.

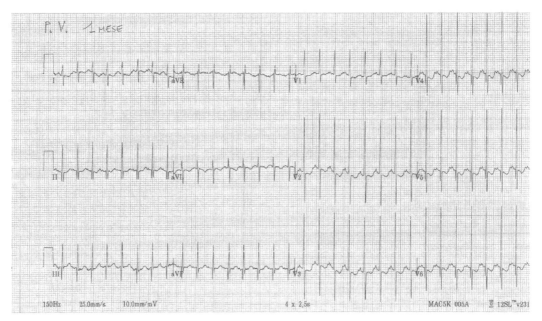

Fig. 4.11 Electrocardiogram recorded of a 1-month-old infant

Looking at the V_1 and V_6 precordial leads in Fig. 4.11, we find that the electrical forces are balanced, which fits the "infant pattern" and is appropriate for the patient's age. In V_1, the R wave of right ventricular depolarization is dominant such that R/S > 1. In V_6, the R wave of left ventricular depolarization is dominant such that R/S > 1. The pathological element in this ECG is the high voltage (3 mV) of the R wave in V_4–V_5–V_6, which is compatible with left ventricular hypertrophy. The QRS frontal axis is normal (+90°).

Ventricular repolarization is normal in V_1–V_2 since the T wave is negative there, but pathological in V_5–V_6 and in the I–aV_L leads, since the T wave is also negative there, suggesting left ventricular overload.

It can be concluded that this is a pathological ECG picture that indicates left ventricular hypertrophy/overload. The patient suffered from a large, hemodynamically significant patent ductus arteriosus.

Biventricular Overload

5

Biventricular overload refers to evidence of volume or pressure overload that involves both ventricles simultaneously. This hemodynamic situation can already be present in newborns as an element of congenital cardiopathies; generally these are more complex such as a complete form of atrioventricular septal defect or have many congenital heart defects associated with them. Alternatively, this situation can appear later on, as a complication following a simpler congenital cardiopathy. Biventricular overload is expressed in an ECG by combined aspects of left and right ventricular hypertrophy.

In practice, the V_1 and V_6 precordial leads should be examined for the following reasons: 1) it is possible to find the prevalent signs of right ventricular hypertrophy, defined in Table 3.1, associated with signs of left ventricular enlargement in V_5 and V_6, such as a high voltage R wave (R > 2.5 mV) or a negative T wave; 2) it is possible to find the prevalent signs of left ventricular hypertrophy, defined in Table 4.1, associated, in V_1, with signs indicating right ventricular enlargement, such as a high voltage R wave (R > 2 mV), or a positive T wave (see Table 5.1).

Table 5.1 Combined ventricular enlargement: combined aspects of left and right ventricular hypertrophy

Signs of left ventricular hypertrophy	combined with	in V_1: R wave > 20 mm (> 2 mV)
		positive T wave
Signs of right ventricular hypertrophy	combined with	in V_5–V_6: R wave > 25 mm (> 2.5 mV)
		negative T wave

M. A. Galli (✉)
Perinatal and Pediatric Cardiology
Ospedale Maggiore Policlinico
Milan, Italy
e-mail: mariellagalli@gmail.com

M. A. Galli, G. B. Danzi, *A Guide to Neonatal and Pediatric ECGs*,
DOI: 10.1007/978-88-470-2856-2_5, © Springer-Verlag Italia 2013

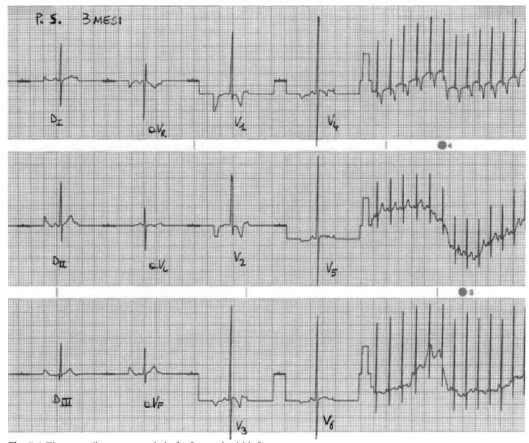

Fig. 5.1 Electrocardiogram recorded of a 3-month-old infant

In the precordial leads of Fig. 5.1, the signs of left ventricular hypertrophy are a 3.2 mV high voltage R wave of left ventricular depolarization in V_5 and V_6, which exceeds the 2.5 mV normal limit. Signs of associated right ventricular hypertrophy are visible in V_1 through a 2.3 mV high voltage R wave of right ventricular depolarization, which exceeds the 2 mV normal limit, and in V_6 through the 15 mm (1.5 mV) deep S wave, which exceeds the 10 mm (1 mV) norm.

The QRS frontal axis is normal at +50°, as is the pattern of ventricular repolarization. The T wave is negative in V_1–V_2 and positive in V_5–V_6.

In this case, the ECG picture is pathological due to signs of combined ventricular enlargement in V_1 and V_6.

The patient suffered from a large, hemodynamically significant perimembranous ventricular septal defect.

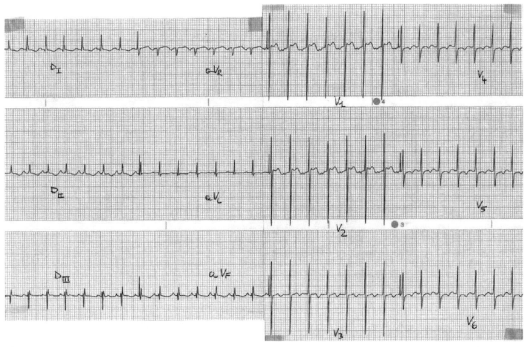

Fig. 5.2 Electrocardiogram recorded of a 6-day-old newborn

Looking at the precordial leads in Fig. 5.2, one can see the "adult pattern" in V_1 since the S wave of left ventricular depolarization is dominant such that R/S < 1. This suggests electrical prevalence of the left ventricle, which is incongruous with the patient's age and indicates left ventricular enlargement; moreover, in V_1 the very deep S wave exceeds the normal limit of 2 mV. In V_6, the R wave of left ventricular depolarization dominates such that R/S > 1, which fits the "infant pattern" and is normal for the patient's age. The +10° left deviated QRS axis is a further sign of left ventricular hypertrophy.

The pattern of ventricular repolarization is pathological. In V_1, the T wave is positive, suggesting right ventricular systolic load. In V_6 and I, the T wave is negative, indicating left ventricular hypertrophy.

In this trace, the prevalent signs of left ventricular enlargement associated with the positive T wave in V_1–V_2 allow for an electrocardiographic diagnosis of combined ventricular enlargement. The patient suffered from a large perimembranous ventricular septal defect with pulmonary artery hypertension.

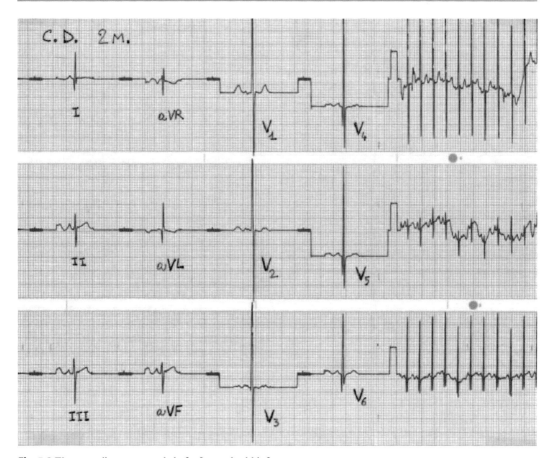

Fig. 5.3 Electrocardiogram recorded of a 2-month-old infant

Looking at the precordial leads in Fig. 5.3, a sign of left ventricular hypertrophy is the high voltage R wave of left ventricular depolarization in V_4 (3.2 mV), V_5 (3.5 mV) and V_6 (2.4 mV). This is confirmed in V_1 by the 23 mm (2.3 mV) S wave of left ventricular depolarization, which exceeds the 20 mm (2 mV) normal limit. In V_1, the R/S > 1 ratio fits the "infant pattern", which is appropriate for the patient's age. The R wave of right ventricular depolarization, however, has an amplitude of 28 mm (2.8 mV), which exceeds the 20 mm (2 mV) normal limit indicating associated right ventricular hypertrophy.

The pathological aspects in ventricular repolarization are the negative T wave in the aV_L lead indicating left ventricular overload, and the positive T wave in V_1–V_2 indicating right ventricular systolic overload. The -30° left deviated QRS axis is a further sign of left ventricle hypertrophy.

The plural elements of left and right ventricular overload in this electrocardiogram compose a picture of combined ventricular enlargement. The patient suffered from a large perimembranous ventricular septal defect with pulmonary artery hypertension.

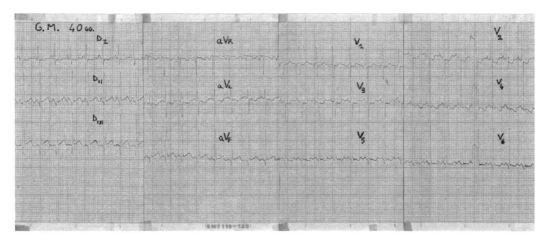

Fig. 5.4 Electrocardiogram recorded of a 40-day-old infant

In Fig. 5.4, at V_1 the morphology of the QRS fits the "infant pattern" since the electrical forces of the right ventricle are dominant and the S wave of left ventricular depolarization is well represented so R/S > 1. This is appropriate for the patient's age. In V_6, the QRS pattern fits the "adult" type since there is no S wave of right ventricular depolarization. This is pathological for the age of the patient and a sign of left ventricular hypertrophy.

The pathological aspects in ventricular repolarization are the negative T wave in the V_5–V_6 leads indicating left ventricular overload and the positive T wave in V_1, which indicates associated right ventricular systolic overload. The +80° QRS frontal axis is normal for the age of the patient.

In this case, the prevalent signs of left ventricular hypertrophy/overload are associated with the positive T wave in V_1, itself a sign of right ventricular overload. Together, they support a diagnosis of combined ventricular enlargement. The patient suffered from a large perimembranous ventricular septal defect.

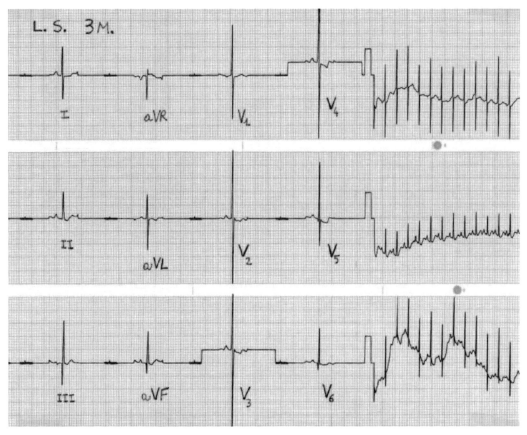

Fig. 5.5 Electrocardiogram recorded of a 3-month-old infant

The considerations made in the ECG in Fig. 5.4 are also valid here (Fig. 5.5). In V_1, the morphology of the QRS complex fits the "infant pattern", which is congruous with the patient's age. In V_6, the QRS pattern fits the "adult" type, which is pathological in relation to the age of the patient and indicates left ventricular hypertrophy.

The pathological aspect of ventricular repolarization is the T wave, which is negative in V_5–V_6 and positive in V_1. This adds information supporting left ventricular overload and associated right ventricular systolic overload. The +90° QRS frontal axis is normal for the patient's age.

In this case as well, the prevalent signs of left ventricular hypertrophy/overload are associated with the positive T wave in V_1, a sign of right ventricular overload, and support a diagnosis of biventricular overload. The patient suffered from the complete form of atrioventricular septal defect.

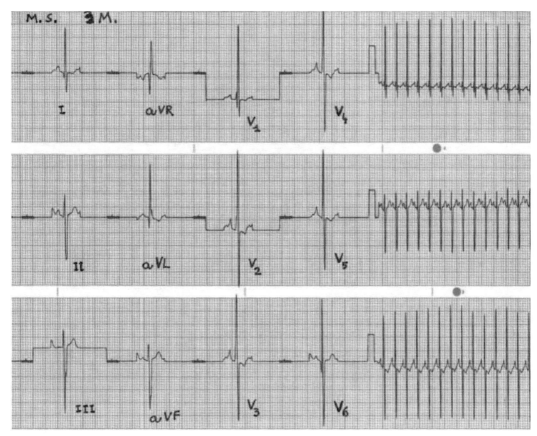

Fig. 5.6 Electrocardiogram recorded of a 3-month-old infant

The signs of right ventricular hypertrophy in the precordial leads (Fig. 5.6) are the pathological 30 mm amplitude of the dominant R wave of right ventricular depolarization in V_1, and the pathological 25 mm (2.5 mV) amplitude of the S wave of right ventricular depolarization in V_6, which exceeds the 10 mm (1 mV) normal limit. In the V_4–V_5–V_6 leads, the voltage of the R wave of left ventricular depolarization is at the 2.5 mV upper limit, suggesting left ventricular hypertrophy.

The morphology of ventricular repolarization in V_1 is pathological since the positive T wave indicates right ventricular systolic overload. The T wave is positive in V_6, which is normal, but negative in the aV_L lateral lead, which indicates left ventricular overload. The −40° left deviated QRS axis is pathological, as is the rule in the type of congenital cardiopathy the patient suffers from.

In this case, the prevalent signs of right ventricular hypertrophy/overload are associated with signs of left ventricular overload. This supports a diagnosis of biventricular overload. The patient suffered from the complete form of atrioventricular septal defect with pulmonary artery hypertension.

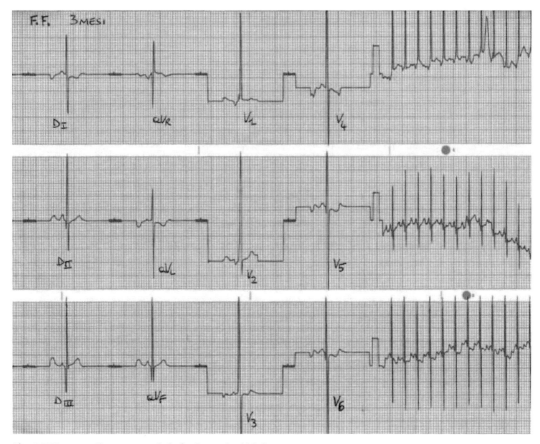

Fig. 5.7 Electrocardiogram recorded of a 3-month-old infant

In Fig. 5.7, the first sign of right ventricular hypertrophy in the V_1 and V_6 precordial leads is the pathological 3.3 mV amplitude of the exclusive R wave of right ventricular depolarization in V_1, which exceeds the 10 mm (1 mV) normal limit. The second is the pathological 3 mV voltage of the S wave of right ventricular depolarization such that R/S < 1 in V_6, which fits the "neonatal pattern" and is incongruous with the patient's age.

The pathological aspect of ventricular repolarization is the positive T wave in V_1, which confirms right ventricular systolic overload. It is negative in V_5–V_6 and DI–aV_L, which adds evidence to the presence of associated left ventricular overload. The +80° QRS frontal axis is within normal limits for the patient's age.

These elements support a diagnosis of combined ventricular enlargement. The patient suffered from a large muscular ventricular septal defect and neonatal repair of aortic coarctation.

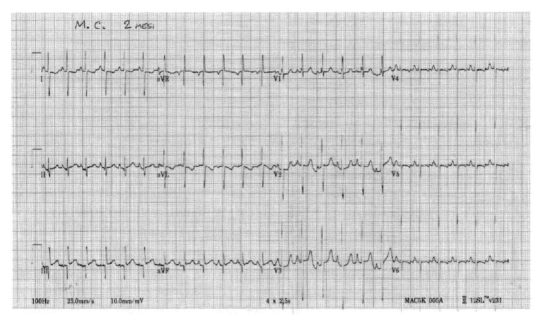

Fig. 5.8 Electrocardiogram recorded of a 2-month-old infant

The pattern of the precordial leads in Fig. 5.8, fits the "infant" type, which is appropriate for the patient's age. Signs of right ventricular hypertrophy, however, are visible in V_6 through a deep S wave of right ventricular depolarization, with a voltage of 27 mm (2.7 mV), which exceeds the normal limit of 10 mm (1 mV). In V_1, the 10 mm voltage of the R wave of right ventricular depolarization is within the norm in that R/S > 1.

The pathological aspect in the electrical activity of ventricular repolarization is the positive T wave in V_1–V_2, which confirms right ventricular systolic overload. The negative T wave in V_5–V_6 and DI–aV_L adds evidence to the presence of associated left ventricular overload. The +100° QRS frontal axis is at the normal limit for the patient's age.

In this case as well, the prevalent signs of right ventricular hypertrophy/overload are associated with the negative T wave in the lateral chest leads, suggesting left ventricular overload. These elements, when combined, support a diagnosis of combined ventricular enlargement. The patient suffered from double-outlet right ventricle with pulmonary artery hypertension.

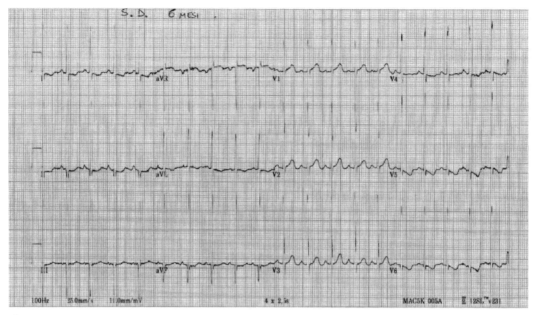

Fig. 5.9 Electrocardiogram recorded of a 6-month-old infant

Looking at the V_1 and V_6 precordial leads (Fig. 5.9), one sees the "adult pattern", which is incongruous with the patient's age, indicating left ventricular hypertrophy. In V_1, the R wave of right ventricular depolarization is well represented at 15 mm but the 25 mm deep S wave of left ventricular depolarization is prevalent so that R/S < 1. The R wave of left ventricular depolarization has a high voltage in V_5 (3.8 mV) and V_6 (3 mV), which exceeds the 2.5 mV normal limit.

The pathological aspect in the electrical activity of ventricular repolarization is the negative T wave in V_5–V_6 and DI–aV_L, supporting evidence for left ventricular overload, and the positive T wave in V_1, supporting evidence for right ventricular systolic overload. The +50° QRS frontal axis is normal for the age of the patient.

In this case, the prevalent signs of left ventricular hypertrophy/overload are associated with the positive T wave in V_1, itself a sign of right ventricular systolic overload. Together, they support a diagnosis of biventricular overload. The patient presented with an echocardiographic picture of dilated cardiomyopathy of the left ventricle, secondary to viral myocarditis.

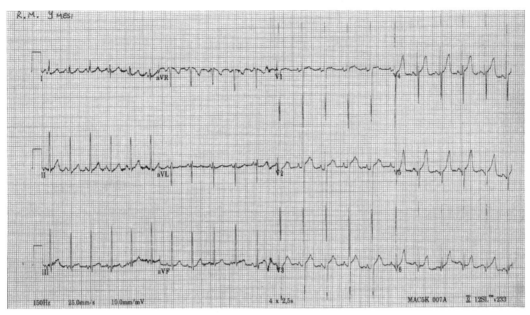

Fig. 5.10 Electrocardiogram recorded of a 9-month-old infant

In Fig. 5.10, the V_6 precordial lead follows the "adult pattern" since the S wave of right ventricular depolarization is absent, and shows left ventricular hypertrophy since there is the high voltage R wave in V_4 (3.2 mV), V_5 (4.5 mV) and V_6 (3.3 mV) with the 2.5 mV deep S wave in the V_1 precordial lead (above the 2mV normal limit). In V_1, the 25 mm (2.5 mV) voltage R wave of right ventricular depolarization exceeds the 2 mV normal limit and this element is compatible with associated right ventricular hypertrophy.

The pathological aspect in the electrical activity of ventricular repolarization is the positive T wave in V_1–V_2, which indicates right ventricular systolic overload. The +80° QRS frontal axis is normal.

Elements of left and right ventricular hypertrophy in this electrocardiogram constitute a picture of combined ventricular enlargement. The patient suffered from a large perimembranous ventricular septal defect with pulmonary artery hypertension.

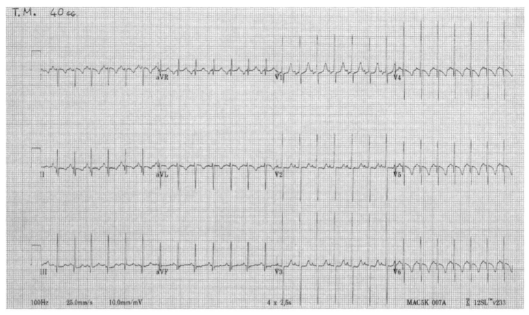

Fig. 5.11 Electrocardiogram recorded of a 40-day-old infant

The pattern of ventricular depolarization seen in V_1 and V_6 of Fig. 5.11 fits the "infant pattern", since the electrical forces of the left and right ventricles are balanced. This is appropriate for the patient's age, and thus, is normal.

The pathological aspects in the electrical activity of ventricular repolarization are the positive T wave in V_1, which indicates right ventricular systolic overload, and the negative T wave in V_5–V_6 and DI–aV_L, which indicates left ventricular overload. The +140° electrical axis of the heart is right deviated.

In this chart, the diagnosis of biventricular overload is based essentially on the pattern of ventricular repolarization. This patient suffered from coarctation of the aorta.

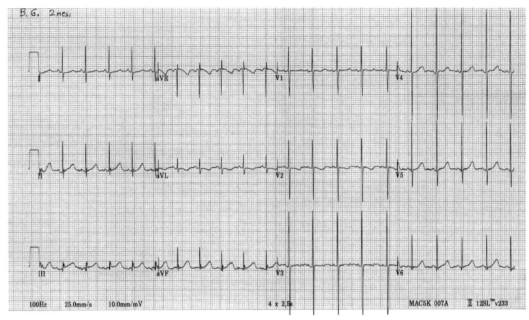

Fig. 5.12 Electrocardiogram recorded of a 2-month-old infant

In V₁, the morphology of the QRS complex fits the "infant pattern", which is appropriate for the patient's age. The R wave of right ventricular depolarization is well represented at 13 mm and the S wave of left ventricular depolarization is the same size so that R/S = 1. V₆ shows an "adult pattern" since the S wave of left ventricular depolarization is absent, which indicates left ventricular hypertrophy, given the patient's age. This is confirmed by the high voltage of the R wave in V₄ (3.2 mV) and V₅ (2.5 mV).

The pathological element in the electrical activity of ventricular repolarization is the positive T wave in V₁. This fact suggests associated right ventricular systolic overload. The positive T wave in V₅–V₆ is normal but is associated with signs of left ventricular hypertrophy and is indicative of left ventricular volume overload. The QRS frontal axis tends toward the left at +40°.

In this case, support for a diagnosis of biventricular overload includes signs of left ventricular hypertrophy associated with the positive T wave in V₁, which suggests right ventricular systolic overload. The patient suffered from a large perimembranous ventricular septal defect with pulmonary artery hypertension.

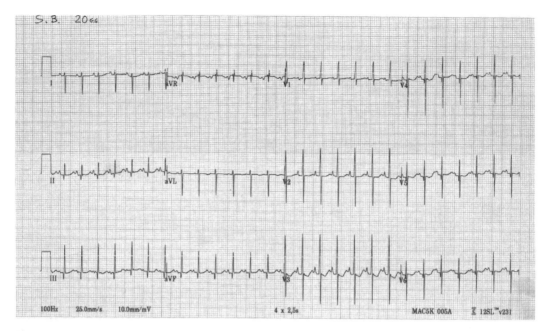

Fig. 5.13 Electrocardiogram recorded of a 20-day-old newborn

Looking at the V_1 and V_6 precordial leads in Fig. 5.13, one can see the "neonatal pattern", which is appropriate for the patient's age and thus, is normal. In V_1, the right ventricle is prevalent such that R/S > 1. In V_6, again the right ventricle is prevalent such that R/S < 1. The QRS frontal axis is right deviated at +130°, which is normal in the first month of life.

Looking at ventricular repolarization, the pathological elements become apparent. In V_1, the positive T wave suggests right ventricular systolic load, while in V_5–V_6 the diphasic T wave suggests left ventricular overload.

In this ECG, the diagnosis of biventricular overload is essentially based on the pathological pattern of ventricular repolarization. The patient suffered from type II truncus arteriosus with stenosis of the right branch of the pulmonary artery.

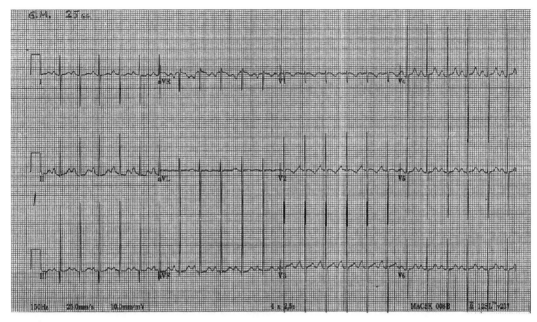

Fig. 5.14 Electrocardiogram recorded of a 25-day-old newborn

Looking at the precordial leads in Fig. 5.14, one can see that the S wave of left ventricular depolarization is dominant in V_1 in that R/S < 0.4. This fits the "adult pattern", which is pathological in relation to this 25-day-old patient's age and supports the diagnosis of left ventricular enlargement. In V_6, the morphology of the QRS complex fits the "neonatal pattern" in that R/S < 1, which is normal for this patient's age. The voltage of the 2.2 mV deep S wave, however, exceeds the 1 mV normal limit (see Table 1.1) and suggests right ventricular enlargement.

The morphology of ventricular repolarization is normal since the T wave is negative in V_1–V_2 and positive in V_5–V_6. The QRS frontal axis is right deviated at +105°, which is also normal for this age.

In summary, this ECG is pathological on account of signs of biventricular enlargement due to volume overload. The patient suffered from a large ostium secundum-type atrial septal defect associated with a mid-sized perimembranous ventricular septal defect and with multiple muscular ventricular septal defects.

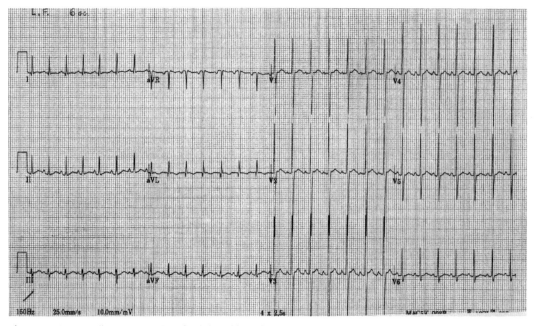

Fig. 5.15 Electrocardiogram recorded of a 6-day-old newborn

In Fig. 5.15, for V_1 the morphology of the QRS complex presents a well represented R wave of right ventricular depolarization at 17 mm. The voltage of the 22 mm deep S wave of left ventricular depolarization, however, supports a diagnosis of left ventricular hypertrophy (see Table 4.1) since it exceeds the 2 mV normal limit.

The morphology of the QRS complex in V_6 is congruous with the "infant pattern", which is normal for a patient this age. The +30° QRS axis is left deviated, which is pathological for the patient's age.

In ventricular repolarization, the positive T wave in V_5–V_6 is normal, but it is negative in the I–aV_L leads, signaling left ventricular overload. The positive T wave in V_1–V_2 suggests associated right ventricular systolic load.

In this case, evidence for a diagnosis of biventricular overload are the signs of left ventricular hypertrophy/overload associated with the positive T wave in V_1–V_2, which suggests right ventricular systolic overload. The patient suffered from transposition of great arteries associated with a large ventricular septal defect.

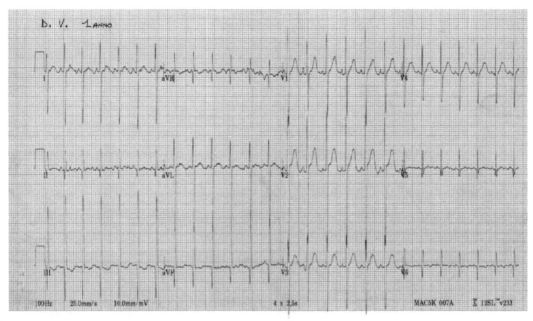

Fig. 5.16 Electrocardiogram recorded of a 12-month-old infant

Looking at the V_1 and V_6 precordial leads in Fig. 5.16, one can see the "adult pattern", which is incongruous with the patient's age and indicates left ventricular hypertrophy. In V_1, the R wave of right ventricular depolarization is well represented at 18 mm but the deep S wave of left ventricular depolarization is pathological due to its 22 mm (2.2 mV) voltage and it is prevalent such that R/S < 1. In V_6, the S wave of right ventricular depolarization is absent.

The deep Q wave, in the III–aV_F extremity leads and in the V_6 lateral chest lead, is a variation of the norm from age 3 months to 3 years. In this case, the 1.6 mV voltage of the Q wave in the III extremity lead points to possible left ventricular hypertrophy.

The pathological aspect of ventricular repolarization is the T wave, which is negative in V_6 and positive in V_1–V_2. This provides useful information to diagnose left ventricular overload and associated right ventricular systolic overload.

The +130° QRS frontal axis is right deviated, which is pathological given the 12-month-old patient's age. In this ECG, evidence to support a diagnosis of biventricular overload is given by the right deviated QRS frontal axis and signs of left ventricular hypertrophy/overload associated with the positive T wave in V_1–V_2, which suggests right ventricular systolic overload. The patient suffered from a large perimembranous ventricular septal defect associated with right ventricular outflow tract obstruction.

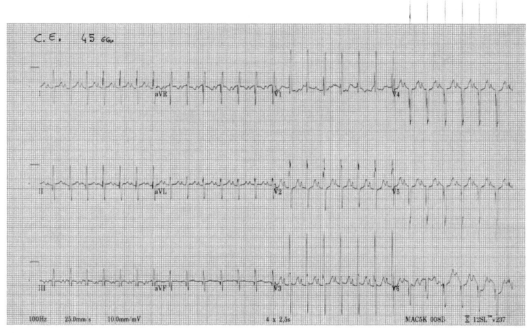

Fig. 5.17 Electrocardiogram recorded of a 45-day-old infant

In Fig. 5.17, the morphology of the QRS, in the V_1 precordial lead, presents a delay in right intraventricular conduction with an rSR' pattern that indicates right ventricular volume overload. The 2 mV high voltage R wave suggests right ventricular hypertrophy. V_6 fits the "infant pattern" in that R/S > 1. The high voltage R wave of left ventricular depolarization in V_4 (4.5 mV), V_5 (3.5 mV) and V_6 (3 mV) is a sign of left ventricular hypertrophy since it exceeds the 2.5 mV normal limit.

The morphology of ventricular repolarization indicates right ventricular systolic load since the T wave is diphasic in V_1 and positive in V_2, which is a pathological sign in the 45-day-old patient. The +80° QRS frontal axis is normal.

In summary, this ECG supports a diagnosis of biventricular pressure and volume overload. The patient suffered from Ebstein's malformation of the tricuspid valve associated with an ostium secundum-type atrial septal defect, with a partial anomalous pulmonary venous drainage of two pulmonary veins in the innominate vein, and with two large muscular ventricular septal defects.

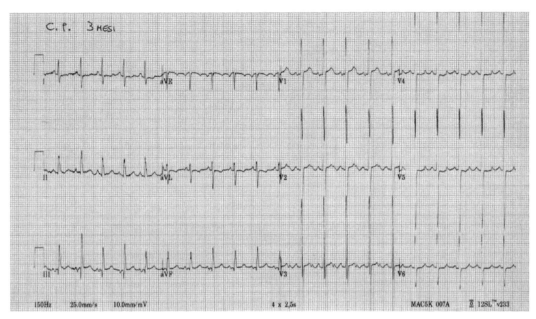

Fig. 5.18 Electrocardiogram recorded of a 3-month-old infant

Looking at the V_1 precordial lead in Fig. 5.18, the dominant S wave of left ventricular depolarization has a high voltage of 3 mV, which exceeds the 2 mV normal limit. The ratio is R/S < 1, showing left ventricular prevalence, which is incongruous with the patient's age and indicates left ventricular enlargement. In V_6, the "infant pattern" is still present since the R wave of left ventricular depolarization is dominant so that R/S > 1, but it shows pathological voltage in V_4 (3.3 mV) and V_5 (3.2 mV), which also suggests left ventricular enlargement.

In terms of ventricular repolarization, there are pathological aspects in V_1–V_2 since the T wave is positive there, indicating right ventricular systolic load. Furthermore, in the V_5–V_6 precordial leads and the I–aV_L leads, the T wave is diphasic, indicating left ventricular overload. The +70° QRS frontal axis is normal.

In this ECG, evidence to support a diagnosis of biventricular overload is given by the prevalent signs of left ventricular hypertrophy/overload accompanied by the positive T wave in V_1–V_2, which indicates right ventricular systolic load. The patient suffered from a large perimembranous ventricular septal defect complicated by pulmonary artery hypertension.

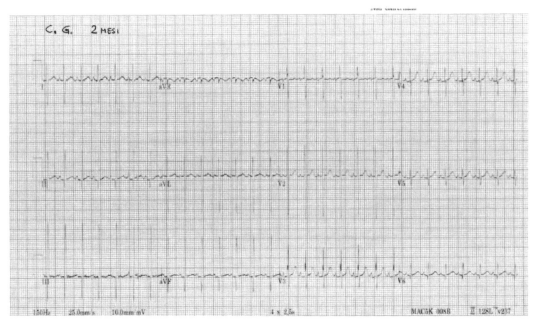

Fig. 5.19 Electrocardiogram recorded of a 2-month-old infant

In Fig. 5.19, one can see the "adult pattern" in the V_1 and V_6 precordial leads, which is incongruous with the patient's age and indicates left ventricular enlargement. In V_1, the R wave of right ventricular depolarization is well represented at 7 mm, but the 10 mm deep S wave of left ventricular depolarization is dominant such that R/S < 1. In V_6, the S wave of right ventricular depolarization is absent. With regard to the morphology of ventricular repolarization, the T wave is positive in V_5–V_6, which is normal. The pathological aspect is that it is also positive in V_1–V_2, indicating right ventricular systolic load. The +120° QRS frontal axis is normal for a patient of this age.

In this ECG, evidence to support a diagnosis of biventricular load is given by signs of left ventricular enlargement accompanied by the positive T wave in V_1–V_2 that indicates right ventricular systolic load. The patient suffered from pulmonary atresia associated with ventricular septal defect.

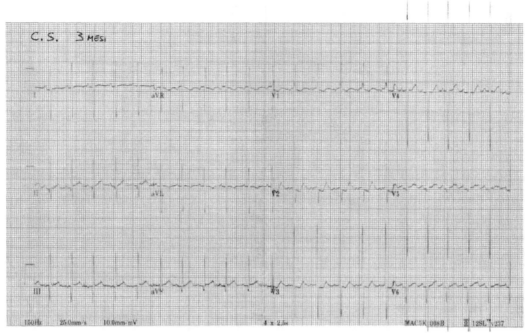

Fig. 5.20 Electrocardiogram recorded of a 3-month-old infant

In this trace (Fig. 5.20), the signs of right ventricular hypertrophy are visible in V_1 through the exclusive 15 mm (1.5 mV) R wave, which exceeds the 1 mV normal limit, and a slight delay in right intraventricular conduction. In V_6, the signs are visible through the deep S wave (2.3 mV) of right ventricular depolarization, which exceeds the 1 mV limit. The high voltage of the R wave of left ventricular depolarization in V_4 (5 mV), V_5 (4 mV) and V_6 (3.5 mV) is a sign of concomitant left ventricular enlargement.

The morphology of ventricular repolarization shows pathological signs in V_1–V_2 since the T wave is diphasic there, suggesting right ventricular systolic load. The +95° QRS frontal axis is normal for a patient this age.

In summary, this is a pathological ECG showing signs of biventricular load. The patient suffered from a large, muscular ventricular septal defect complicated by pulmonary artery hypertension.

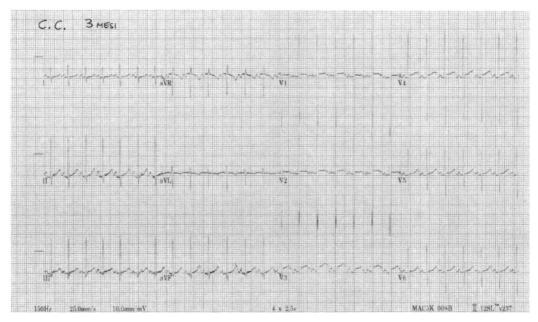

Fig. 5.21 Electrocardiogram recorded of a 3-month-old infant

In Fig. 5.21, for V_1, the 22 mm R wave of right ventricular depolarization is well represented, but the 27 mm S wave of left ventricular depolarization is dominant such that R/S < 1. The S wave is pathological due to its 2.7 mV voltage, which exceeds the 2 mV normal limit. This is incongruous with the age of the patient and indicates left ventricular hypertrophy. The morphology of the QRS complex in V_6 fits the "infant pattern", which is normal for a patient this age.

With regards to ventricular repolarization, a pathological aspect is the positive T wave in V_1–V_2, which indicates right ventricular systolic load. In V_5–V_6, the positive T wave is normal, but in this context, it confirms left ventricular volume overload. The +80° QRS frontal axis is normal for a patient this age.

In this ECG, evidence to support a diagnosis of biventricular load is given by the prevalent signs of left ventricular enlargement associated with signs of right ventricular systolic load (positive T wave in V_1–V_2). The patient suffered from a large perimembranous ventricular septal defect complicated by pulmonary artery hypertension in Down's syndrome.

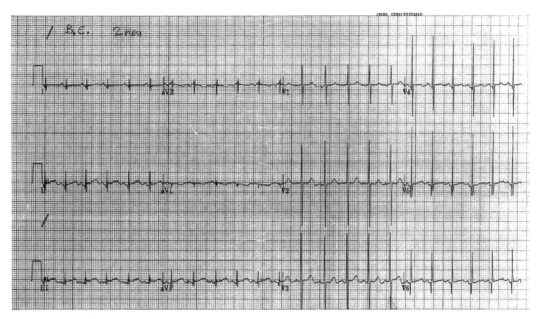

Fig. 5.22 Electrocardiogram recorded of a 2-month-old infant

In V_1 of Fig. 5.22, the morphology of the QRS complex fits that of the "infant pattern" since the 10 mm R wave of right ventricular depolarization is well represented and the 10 mm S wave of left ventricular depolarization is equal to it, such that R/S = 1. In V_6, the situation fits the "adult pattern" since the S wave of right ventricular depolarization is absent. This is pathological in relation to the patient's age and indicates left ventricular enlargement, which is also confirmed by the high voltage (2.5 mV) of the R wave in V_4 and V_5.

The pathological aspect in ventricular repolarization is the positive T wave in V_1–V_2. This adds information to a diagnosis of associated right ventricular systolic overload. The positive T wave in V_5–V_6 is normal but associated with signs of left ventricular hypertrophy, and indicative of left ventricular volume overload. The +75° QRS frontal axis is normal.

In this case, evidence to support a diagnosis of biventricular overload is given by the prevalent signs of left ventricular enlargement associated with the positive T wave in V_1–V_2, which indicate right ventricular systolic overload. The patient suffered from a large perimembranous ventricular septal defect with pulmonary artery hypertension in Down's syndrome.

Part III
Miscellaneous ECGs

Miscellaneous ECGs

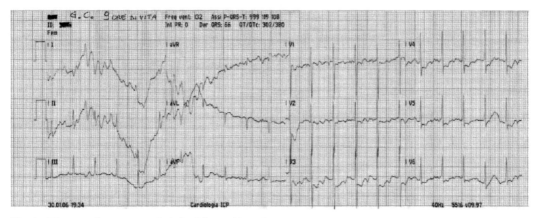

6

Fig. 6.1 Electrocardiogram recorded of a 9-hour-old newborn

The pathological element here (Fig. 6.1), is the morphology of ventricular repolarization. In the V_3–V_4–V_5 and V_6 precordial leads, one can see an ST depression of about 3 mm, which indicates myocardial ischemia.

This newborn suffered from a transient myocardial ischemia with severe perinatal hypoxia.

M. A. Galli (✉)
Perinatal and Pediatric Cardiology
Ospedale Maggiore Policlinico
Milan, Italy
e-mail: mariellagalli@gmail.com

M. A. Galli, G. B. Danzi, *A Guide to Neonatal and Pediatric ECGs*,
DOI: 10.1007/978-88-470-2856-2_6, © Springer-Verlag Italia 2013

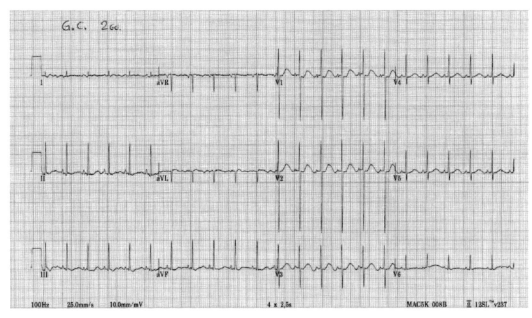

Fig. 6.2 Electrocardiogram recorded of a 2-day-old newborn

This trace (Fig. 6.2) was registered to the same patient as that in Fig. 6.1, but at 2 days old.

Here, one can see that the morphology of ventricular repolarization in the precordial leads has completely normalized.

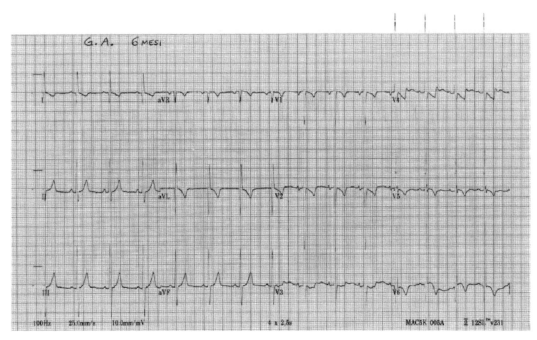

Fig. 6.3 Electrocardiogram recorded of a 6-month-old infant

The important element in this trace (Fig. 6.3) is the deep Q wave in the I–aV$_L$ leads and the V$_6$ lateral chest lead. It is pathological due to its width at 40 ms, and its voltage of 0.8 mV in V$_6$ and 1.5 mV in aV$_L$, which indicate myocardial necrosis. Associated with this are ischemic alterations in ventricular repolarization, and T-wave inversion in the left precordial leads reflects myocardial ischemia.

This trace fits the "infant pattern" which is appropriate for the patient's age. There are, however, signs of left ventricular enlargement: the high voltage R wave of left ventricular depolarization, which goes up to 4 mV in V$_4$, V$_5$ and V$_6$.

In summary, the ECG is pathological due to signs of myocardial necrosis in the lateral chest lead, associated with signs of left ventricular enlargement. The patient presented with a dilated cardiomyopathy of the left ventricle, secondary to myocardial ischemia, caused by the anomalous origin of the left coronary artery from the main pulmonary artery.

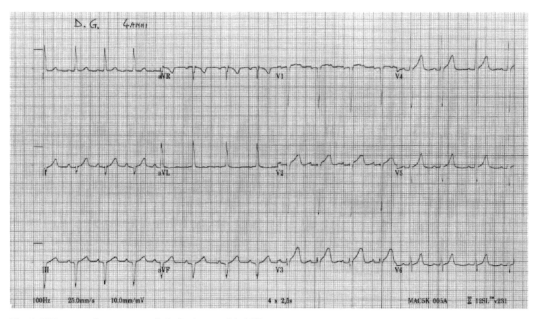

Fig. 6.4 Electrocardiogram recorded of a 4-year-old child

An important characteristic in this ECG (Fig. 6.4) is the presence of QS in V_1 and the absence of the Q wave in the left V_5 and V_6 precordial leads. This is an inversion of the normal septal depolarization pattern, an electrical situation of discordant atrioventricular connection. This ventricular inversion means that both the right and left surfaces of the ventricular septum and the left and right branches of the conduction pathway are inverted. In a normal heart, the electrical activation of the common ventricular myocardium always begins in the left subendocardial region of the ventricular septum. It is directed forward from left to right because the right ventricle is anterior. In the discordant atrioventricular connection, however, the left ventricle is anterior with respect to the right one, so the electrical forces are directed backward from the left side of the septum to the right. This explains why the QRS is initially negative in V_1 and positive in V_6. This patient had a corrected congenital transposition of the great arteries.

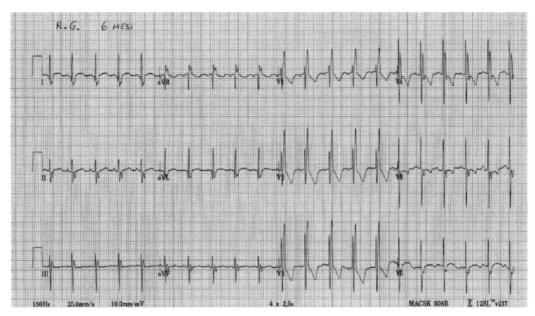

Fig. 6.5 Electrocardiogram recorded of a 6-month-old infant

This ECG (Fig. 6.5) shows a QRS duration of 100 ms, which exceeds the normal limit of 80 ms. The rSR' type morphology of the QRS complex in V_1 indicates a complete right bundle branch block.

The patient presented with the results of a surgical repair of a large perimembranous ventricular septal defect. In fact, the complete right bundle branch block is a typical result expected in cardiac surgery that requires patch applications to close ventricular septal defects or right ventricular incision.

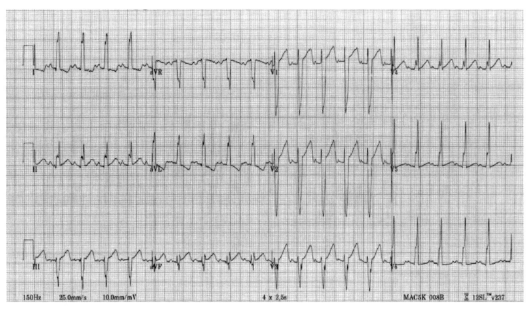

Fig. 6.6 Electrocardiogram recorded of an 11-month-old infant

This trace (Fig. 6.6) shows a QRS duration of 100 ms, which exceeds the normal limit of 80 ms. The morphology of the QRS complex in I–aV$_L$ and V$_1$–V$_6$ indicates a complete left bundle branch block. The patient suffered from dilated cardiomyopathy of the left ventricle resulting from viral myocarditis. A complete left bundle branch block always indicates a severe myocardial pathological condition.

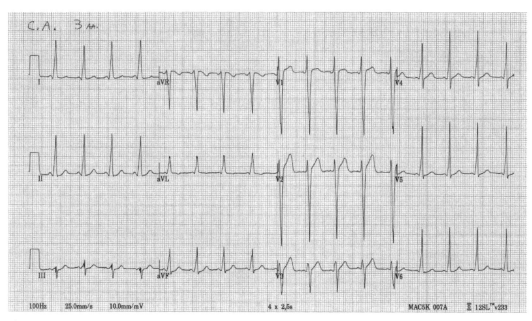

Fig. 6.7 Electrocardiogram recorded of a 3-year-old child

This trace (Fig. 6.7) shows a short (60 ms) PR interval, which is below the normal range for a patient this age (from 100 to 160 ms). This element is associated with an elongated 100 ms QRS complex, which was deformed by the delta wave of ventricular preexcitation. The QRS frontal axis is directed toward the left at +30°. The patient suffered from ventricular preexcitation.

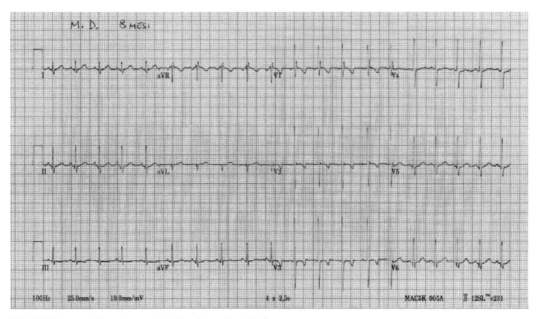

Fig. 6.8 Electrocardiogram recorded of an 8-month-old infant

This ECG (Fig. 6.8) fits the "infant pattern", which is appropriate for the age of this patient. In the V_1 precordial lead, the morphology of the QRS is RSr' type in that R > r' and QRS length is 60 ms, which is within the 80 ms normal limit. The elements constitute a simple right intraventricular conduction delay, which generally carries no pathological significance when it presents with R > r'. In fact, at the echocardiography, the patient presented with a completely normal heart.

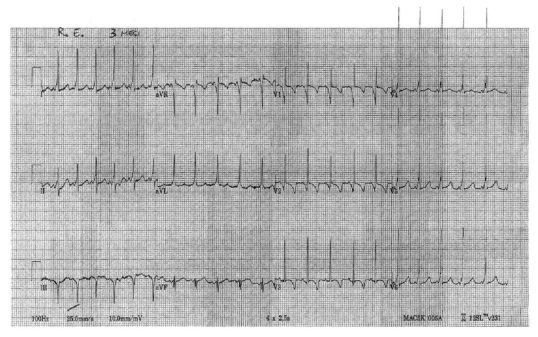

Fig. 6.9 Electrocardiogram recorded of a 3-month-old infant

This ECG (Fig. 6.9) shows a short, 60 ms PR interval, which falls below the normal range of 80 ms to 140 ms for the age of this patient. This element is associated with an elongated 90 ms QRS, which is deformed by the delta wave of ventricular preexcitation, especially in V_1 and V_2. The QRS frontal axis is left deviated. In this case, the electrocardiographical diagnosis is ventricular preexcitation.

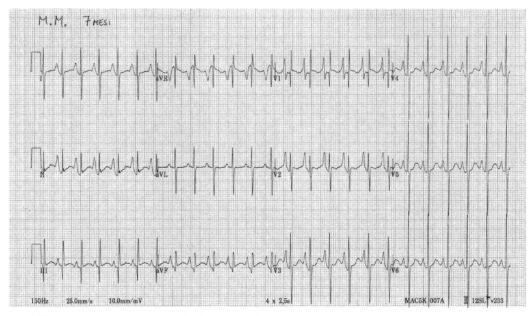

Fig. 6.10 Electrocardiogram recorded of a 7-month-old infant

This ECG (Fig. 6.10) shows monstrous P waves of atrial depolarization with a voltage of up to 0.7 mV, which exceeds the 0.25 mV normal limit. This indicates right atrial enlargement. Furthermore, the PR interval is prolonged to 150 ms, which exceeds the 140 ms limit for this age and indicates first degree atrioventricular block.

The morphology of ventricular depolarization in the precordial leads fits the "infant pattern", which is appropriate for the age of the patient. An incomplete right bundle branch block with rSR' pattern is also visible in V_1. The patient suffered from severe Ebstein's malformation of the tricuspid valve.

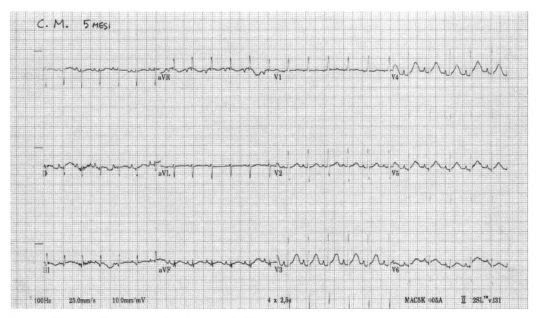

Fig. 6.11 Electrocardiogram recorded of a 5-month-old infant

The salient characteristic of this trace is the +180° right hyperdeviated QRS frontal axis (Fig. 6.11). Looking at the morphology of the V_1 and V_6 precordial leads, one can see the "neonatal pattern" since the right ventricle is dominant. This is inappropriate for a patient of this age. In V_1, the exclusive R wave has a voltage of 0.7 mV, which is at the limit of the norm for this age. In V_6, the S wave is dominant such that R/S < 1.

On the electrocardiogram, both of these elements point to Noonan's syndrome. The patient suffered from moderate pulmonary valve stenosis and Noonan's syndrome. There are electrocardiographic aspects that are typical of Noonan's syndrome and unrelated to the severity of pulmonary valve stenosis.

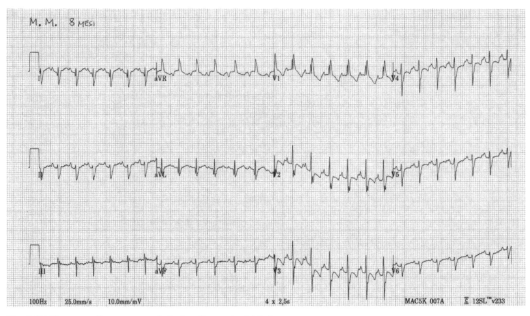

Fig. 6.12 Electrocardiogram recorded of an 8-month-old infant

As in the last ECG, one can see a +220° right hyperdeviated QRS frontal axis (Fig. 6.12). In the morphology of the precordial leads, one can see a complete right bundle branch block in V_1. In V_6, the S wave is dominant such that R/S < 1.

The patient suffered from mild pulmonary valve stenosis and Noonan's syndrome. There are electrocardiographic aspects that are typical of Noonan's syndrome and unrelated to the severity of pulmonary valve stenosis.

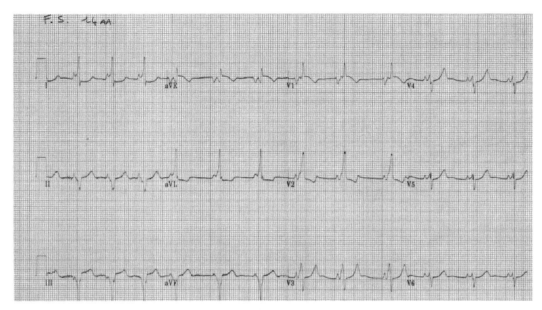

Fig. 6.13 Electrocardiogram recorded of a 14-year-old girl

The salient characteristic in this ECG is the short, 80 ms PR interval, which falls below the normal range of 120–220 ms for the age of the patient (Fig. 6.13). This aspect is associated with an elongated, 120 ms QRS, which was deformed by the delta wave of ventricular preexcitation.

The leftward and superior QRS frontal axis at −70°, and R/S < 1 in V_6, are characteristic of the electrocardiographic picture of Noonan's syndrome. The patient suffered from Noonan's syndrome, moderate pulmonary valve stenosis and ventricular preexcitation.

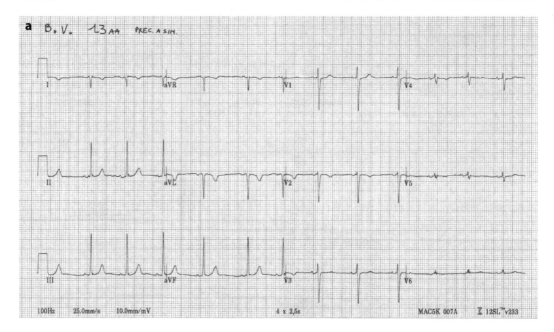

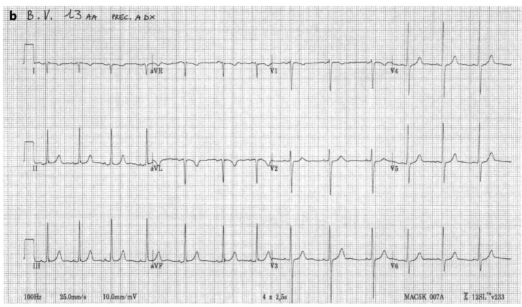

Fig. 6.14 a,b Two electrocardiograms recorded of the same 13-year-old girl

In Fig. 6.14a, the precordial leads are positioned on the left hemithorax. In Fig. 6.14b, they are positioned on the right hemithorax. In this case, the normal morphology of the QRS in the right precordials leads indicates dextrocardia.

In the extremity leads the P-wave deflection is positive in aV_R but negative in aV_L and this suggests inverted atria and indicates atrial situs inversus. The patient suffered from Kartagener's syndrome with visceral situs inversus, atrial situs inversus and dextrocardia, with no associated cardiac defects.

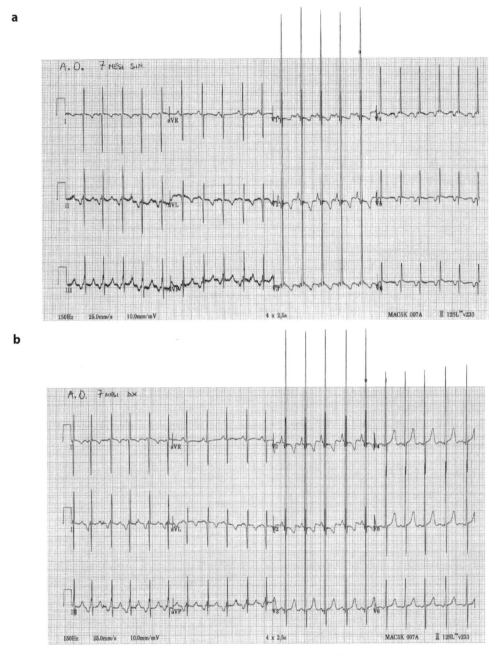

Fig. 6.15 a,b Two electrocardiograms recorded of the same 7-month-old infant

In Fig. 6.15a, the precordial leads are positioned in the left hemithorax. In Fig. 6.15b, they are positioned in the right hemithorax. The morphology of the QRS in the right precordial leads indicates dextrocardia and right ventricular hypertrophy due to the high voltage of the R wave, that reaches up to 6 mV.

In the extremity leads, the P-wave deflection is negative in II, III and aV_F extremity leads, but positive in aV_R; this indicates coronary sinus rhythm. The patient suffered from dextrocardia with a morphologically right univentricular heart.